STRONGER
THAN CANCER

Take Action Today, Beat the Odds and Start Living Your Life

BY
LYN CIKARA

Lyn Cikara
Portland, OR

Copyright © 2017 Lyn Cikara

Download free healing visualization audio at: https://lyncikara.com/publications/

DEDICATION

To my dearest friend and soul mate, Skattie. You taught me how to live and how to laugh.

To my five daughters, Lauren, Samantha, Melissa, Megan and Sarah-Jane. You continue to push me to reach beyond what I think is possible.

TABLE OF CONTENTS

Dedication 3

Acknowledgments 6

Introduction 8

Chapter 1: Decide to Live...12

Chapter 2: The Four Pillars of Healing.......................35

SECTION 1: MIND...38

Chapter 3: Emotions 39

    Sad..42

    Mad 48

    Bad 53

    Scared 56

    Glad..57

Chapter 4: Mindset 64

Chapter 5: Plan to Live Consciously............................71
  Visualization and guided imagery.....................72
  Writing and drawing....................................76

Chapter 6: Choose your team of healers consciously.......82

Chapter 7: Consciously Choose Your Environment...........92

SECTION 2: BODY......................................102

Chapter 8: Your Body...................................103
  Three healing options to explore....................106
    Medical..106
    Wellness approaches................................109
    Movement...113

SECTION 3: SPIRIT....................................117

Chapter 9: Spirit......................................118
  Finding your purpose.................................122
  Spiritual practices..................................124

SECTION 4: SUPPORT...................................138

Chapter 10: Your Support System........................139

Choose...141

What to look for.......................................145

Be explicit about how to support you...................149

Conclusion...152

About the Author.......................................155

ACKNOWLEDGMENTS

My healing journey began because I was given a book. In spite of suggestions to read books about healing, I had little interest in looking at or hearing another thing about cancer. However, there was a book that changed all that for me, *Love, Medicine and Miracles,* by Dr. Bernie Siegel. Reading has contributed to my life and ability to continue living. This book is a result of many authors' contributions to the knowledge about living life with and beyond cancer. These authors include Louise Hay, Andrew Weil, Jeff Kane, Simonton & Simonton, Kim Dalzell and Christine Horner and numerous writers in the field of self-mastery, emotional intelligence, leadership and success.

There have been significant influencers in my life who have contributed to the insights and knowledge I have gained on the topic of living beyond cancer. Some of these influencers have no idea of the impact their words and wisdom have had on my survival. These influencers include David and Jane Wimbush, Eileen Lindsay, Skattie's husband, Jürgen and their three children Katherine, Peter and Rebecca.

The physicians in my life who were true healers: You supported me and you supported my outrageous ideas about healing cancer. Dr. S.J. Lachmann, Dr. Harley Yoder, Dr. Elliott, Dr. Mark Hollemon, Dr. Rafat Ansari, Dr. Kasra Karimalou, Dr. Alison Conlin and Dr. Tori Hudson.

My cardiac magician, acupuncturist and Chinese herbal genius, Kjell Moline and my wholeness coach Jeanette Broneé. You both are my life saviors.

The people who contributed to the production of this book: Chandler Bolt, my buddy Gina Indigo, my coach Scott Allen and my editor, Nina Silberstein, a cancer survivor herself, and the Self Publishing School group. A huge thank you for keeping me on track and showing me the possibility.

The champions of this book are the people whose stories have touched my life and whose lives have filled me with faith and wonder. You know who you are. Thank you for living your lives as whole human beings.

My five daughters who have helped me grow in knowledge and have given me the support, courage and determination to get me this far. I love you.

Thank you all for helping to make this book a reality.

INTRODUCTION

This book is about giving you hope so that the fear of cancer and its outcomes will subside and the life you have to live becomes about living again. I won't proclaim any cures, just remind you of common sense ways to think of your life and what you want from it in spite of having a diagnosis of cancer. I will share my story of survival and learning, and share what I think will be useful ideas to help you establish the path you want to live successfully with hope and joy for your future again.

One of the biggest problems with being diagnosed with cancer is that it makes every negative story, headline and fact about cancer jump out at you and becomes the focus of your attention. There is so much negative data to prove that things will not turn out well. The media are not helpful in boosting confidence. On the contrary, they add to your fears. My solution is to put the data and bad news into perspective for you. I thought I would start my book with some good data for you to think about: Did you know that *the number of people **living beyond a cancer** diagnosis reached nearly 14.5 million in 2014 and is expected to rise to almost 19 million by 2024?* This is a direct quote from the National Cancer Institute of America website (www.cancer.gov.). Its estimation made early in 2016 was that 1.7 million new cases of cancer would be diagnosed in the U.S. An estimate of deaths from cancer for 2016 is only a fraction of the total expected new diagnoses for the same year. That means that the vast majority of people diagnosed with cancer survive.

The headlines do not tell us these facts; instead, we hear only about the death rate. This sensational reporting successfully impresses upon us the anticipation of the worst outcome when a loved one or we are diagnosed with cancer. But it is not true! The bottom line – more people *survive* cancer than die from it every year.

This diagnosis seems to make us, the people living with the disease and our loved ones, targets for horror stories about the disease's prowess from every angle. We are told more urban legends, more community stories and personal experiences of how cancer has destroyed lives rather than stories about survival against these odds.

Say the word "cancer" and dread is etched into the faces around you. We have all been conditioned to expect the worst even though we hear platitudes like, "You've got this" and "You'll be just fine," "You can beat this," with no conviction in the voices of the people making these statements. **I'm here to tell you that these dooming data and stories hide the real truth of survival and success when having to deal with cancer.**

There are strong stories of hope, notwithstanding significant odds, that I want you to hear about so that your belief system changes. There *is* a way to live life fully with hope regardless of a diagnosis of cancer.

I have been diagnosed with cancer three times and it hasn't beaten me yet. The first time was twenty-seven years ago, then ten years ago and, most recently, three years ago. My first diagnosis was of metastatic breast cancer with eleven positive lymph nodes removed during surgery. My predicted survival rate was not great because the cancer had already spread by the time I was diagnosed. Ten years ago I was re-diagnosed. That time there were tumors in my lung and my liver. I survived. Three years ago it came back. This time it was found in fluid that had settled in my lungs and around my heart, causing pericarditis, which landed me in hospital and led to the third cancer diagnosis.

Still, here I am to tell you that there is hope. I beat cancer three times and I am going to share how I did it, so you can beat what cancer is trying to do to you, too.

After watching me survive the first bout of cancer, my general practitioner said to me a long time ago that he believed that I had "found the cure." I believe I have found the key to survival notwithstanding any diagnosis and I'm going to share this with you so that you can, too. In this book I will tell you some simple practices that you and your loved ones can start right away to help you fight the cancer, overcome the fear and live a full life. You will learn how to "live life loudly" and feel empowered against cancer right away.

The data we do not hear about is that more people survive cancer than die from it. The stories we hear limit the truth because sensation and fear sell. The stories I will tell are personal ones to give you the tools to be successful and live life fully again.

Chapter 1

DECIDE TO LIVE

~

The biggest personal challenge for us, after diagnosis, is what to do with our fear of death, loss and suffering. In this chapter I will show you how making a simple but definite decision about your life is, in itself, life-giving. I will introduce you to my three experiences with cancer and how I stumbled on this truth; also how it influenced others to outlive predictions of imminent doom.

My belief is that the way to regain control of the fears brought on by cancer is to start thinking about what is important to you about your life. Fearing death won't get you to living life fully again.

The most important step to take towards surviving cancer is to make a decision about life. Your decision doesn't have to be a bold, loud declaration of your cure or the path you will follow; all it has to be is a decision about what you want from life.

This might seem strange to you right now when you are facing the reality of death more acutely than ever before. Life is what you have right now; you have to try to understand the meaning of that in order to make your decision about life. Not death. The reality of being diagnosed with cancer is that you are forced to look at death. If you remain there and only dwell on death, life will slip away without you noticing life in the interim. Knowing why you are alive, knowing why you want to continue to live and knowing why your life has meaning are the core of your motivation to continue to live.

Take a moment and complete this sentence, "I want to live life to the fullest because..."

My reason for living after being diagnosed with cancer the first time was that I had five young daughters and I could not imagine their lives without their mother. Even though it was with shaky uncertainty at that time, I decided to live. I started out bargaining with life to give me enough years to see my one-year-old grow up and turn twenty one. Imagining her twenty-first birthday, handing over the traditional "key to the door" ended in my imagining me keeling over and dying right there. What an awful birthday present! So, instead, I have decided to live way beyond my daughters' life events. My life is here for me to live. It is that simple.

You might not have any children or significant people in your life to live for. The importance of this exercise is to understand that you are living your life for you. Dig deep to find what makes you want to live. What things do you want to do, see and what experiences have you not had yet? If your life has not had much meaning up to now, this is the time to start the search for meaning.

I met a young woman through my niece in South Africa years ago. This woman who confided in my niece that she had advanced cancer, was not doing well with the chemo and had not told her mother about the cancer. My niece and she were work colleagues in a call center where they had little chance of interacting because of their work set-up. Gina (a fictitious name I gave her) took advantage of the anonymity of the workplace to stay undiscovered in her struggles even though she had told my niece little snippets of what was going on. My niece had experience with my cancer and didn't ever see me isolating myself, so she thought it was important for Gina to talk to someone about what she was going through and to get real support. She was able to get Gina to agree to a long-distance call from me.

The biggest reason for Gina's isolation was that her mother had staunchly hidden her true emotions about her own divorce from her children. She tightly guarded against showing any emotions. Gina grew up feeling the distance between her mother and herself as meaning that her mother did not really care about Gina. During her illness, Gina's interpretation was that when you were suffering, you showed strength by keeping the stiff upper lip and not burdening others with your struggles. What she saw whenever she went to the hospital for her treatment reinforced this notion. People kept to themselves, absorbed in their worlds, not letting others in. What I discovered about Gina was that underlying this stoicism was a silent scream to be heard!

We talked several times about her true needs from life; what a good life would look like. Most of her answers were "I don't know" or "I don't care." One time I asked her whether the rest of her life, as she saw it, would include her mother. Suddenly after that question, our calls stopped. My niece told me that Gina had resigned from her job and had disappeared. Several years later Gina reached out to my niece with a simple explanation: She had decided to live. Working in a cubicle cut off from others wasn't the life she had envisioned for herself. She called her mother and told her exactly what the status of her illness was and what she thought her mother's expectations were for her behavior. She told her mother that she had chosen to go through the most severe of chemo treatments and that it would probably kill her. Gina was blown away when her mother showed her the warmth and compassion she thought was impossible to expect. Her mother was at her side through all her treatments and hospitalizations. Gina's telling me that she didn't care about life wasn't true, she did care and she did live. She thought that she had found reasons why she didn't care and in telling her mother that, she discovered a world of caring that helped her to continue to live.

When deciding to live, it is a decision to embrace life, not hold onto it. Although I had my naïve initial dialogue of why and how long I would live, I was also aware of the ever-present thought of death. At that time, I had no idea of how to deal with either. Now I know that the details didn't really matter; the decision to live did.

We all have to die. Cancer puts death onto the radar for us earlier than expected. That doesn't mean that there is a predictable time or pathway to death, no matter what the media and medical predictions tell us. There are many stories about survival far beyond life-expectancy predictions of doctors. You can be that miracle, too.

Life is a miracle. We know this through the joy we experience at the birth of a new baby. The hard, clinical fact of a newborn is that this little infant will grow up and die. What do we focus on when a baby is born? We focus on dreams and aspirations, of a life yet to be lived. What if, at every milestone we gave up on the dreams and aspirations, because death is surely getting closer? That is not how we live! We celebrate birthdays every year with joy and love, focusing on life and more living. Why is it, then, that a milestone of a certain diagnosis robs us of that joy and hope? We give it undeserved power over us and that is what leads to death - the death of our spirit of hope. Choose to live and to celebrate every day of life.

I have always held the opinion that doctors and statistics do not define me. They shouldn't define you either. Decide now what you believe about your life. Write it down. This is a good time to tell you to start a journal. There will be many times that I give you exercises to write or draw, so find a journal that smells and feels good to you and start writing things and thoughts down. Start with defining why you live. Remember, we do not live for others we live for ourselves.

When I thought of my children growing up without me, I was not sad for them, I was really sad for myself. I was sad that it was difficult to see a future for myself with the outcomes being implied by the diagnosis. I still wanted to do so much in life! I am a stubborn person. When given a story about my life that I cannot believe, I rebel and set out to disprove or change the story. I usually make these decisions without a foggy clue of how I will accomplish them. So far, it has served me, and others I have encountered with cancer well. Decide WHY. You don't need to know HOW just now, but be open to possibilities. A powerful reason *why* you want to live will help you define *how* you will live. Do not let the thought of being "terminal" deter you. All life is terminal. Now start living again!

I have a powerful story about a bold decision, made by an incredible woman that changed her life and inspired me. This is a story of hope and encouragement for all of us. In 2014 I received a work email announcing the news that a colleague, who I did not know personally at that time, was taking a leave of absence due to sudden and severe illness. Concerned whispers around the company were for everyone to send prayers and good thoughts her way because she had cancer and things "were not good." People tend to skirt the topic but continue to talk about others and their fate behind their backs. I like to hear it straight from the source, ask questions and see if I can offer something in return. I prefer to have all "cancer talk" out in the open, not in hushed whispers, so I wrote a card to the woman, encouraging her not to give up, telling her a little about my story and inviting her to call me if she wanted to talk. Within an hour of her opening the mail she called. First she poured out the whole story and the details of her doctors telling her the severity of her Stage 4 cancer and their opinion that she should put her affairs in order because they predicted that she would not see the end of summer. It was May when I heard her story. After listening to her, I asked her what she thought about what the doctors' predictions for her life. Her energy rose to a completely different level when she said that she wanted to live! She spoke about the life she wanted to live and what she wanted to do and accomplish. She spoke with passion about having a family and being too young to die. It was almost as though I had given her permission to dream again. She wanted to live! There was so much passion in that decision!

After making that decision to live, came many more decisions she had to make. None were easy, but her drive and reason to live gave her the stamina to make the hard decisions and to live by them. She and her husband embarked on the most impressive hunt for the right treatments, diets and surgeries. She changed her diet and her lifestyle, they chose and rejected medical approaches and went on hikes and holidays to explore places they had always wanted to see. She became the most dedicated survivor I have ever encountered. Her fervor and knowledge became an inspiration for me. At the time of her three-month scans to review any progress that may have been made, there were signs of bone growth where there had been bone cancer previously! There were other significant signs of tumors shrinking or disappearing that gave her the impetus to continue to fight every way that she could.

This incredible woman has become my role model for never giving up. She has continued to live a wonderful life, filled with joy and energy for every day. Her story is miracle of life and three years later, she is still alive with a little boy whose first birthday she and her husband celebrated this past December.

How do you think it is possible that, given three months to live can turn into three years of life? By her simple decision to live, to search for her cure and her focus, and a dedication to nothing else but to live, she has done more than survive. L'Chaim! To Life, my friend!

Make a decision that you can believe in and devote yourself to that decision. Life follows.

Going through cancer treatment is not an easy journey to choose. I believe the drive behind the challenges are what help us survive in spite of feeling physically weak and depleted at times. Making a clear decision and focusing on that is the key to making it through anything that we have to face with cancer. Life seems to test us along the way at all times. A clear focus and a fearless declaration of our focus do help. My friend did not do this alone; she had the support of her family and friends who were there to cheer her on, hug and cry with her when she needed to, and to celebrate when there were anniversaries and the birth of a baby.

The decision to live may involve much smaller decisions that can become symbols of turning your back on cancer. Not everything is a grand event when dealing with cancer. When I was diagnosed the second time I was truly addicted to sugar and struggled to live without it. My nutritionists had both strongly suggested that sugar had to disappear from my diet. At the clinic where I was working people were constantly bringing in gifts of chocolates, cookies, cake and ice cream. I would dig into the goodies with great enjoyment daily. During a PET scan soon after my diagnosis, I learned that the method used to reveal cancer cells was to inject a glucose-based isotope into my veins to help the cancer cells show up on the scan. I was told that only working muscle and cancer held onto the glucose long enough to show up on the scan. That was when the reality that cancer feeds off sugar hit me pretty hard. At that point I had decided that life still held great importance for me, the insight about sugar helped me cut out all sugar "cold turkey" and keep it out of my diet for many years.

My decision to live overshadowed my cravings for sugar. My *why* helped me when I needed to find a *how*.

Just recently, I had been struggling with a sense of fear that the cancer had come back and that it was causing a downward spiral in my overall health. This situation had persisted for a couple of months without anyone in the medical field having definitive answers for me. None of the tests indicated any cancer; however, because the symptoms persisted, my "cancer brain" reared its ugly head and started convincing me that cancer was taking over again. During this time, in one of his classes, my yoga instructor, who is an incredibly intuitive person, suggested visualizing a significant person reaching out and touching our hearts. My visualization surprised me. It was of my dearest friend and soul mate, Skattie, who had died many years ago of leukemia. Seeing her reaching towards me fired up an enormous desire to be with her. That longing was so intense that it made me think that I wanted to die to be with her.

The temptation to give up was huge and it scared me. The shock that I experienced by having a desire to die was immense. Along with the shock came the revelation that the thought of giving up and accepting death was not something I was ready for. I had too much life in me! Fear had gnawed at the way I was living my life, to the point of almost believing that this might *be it*.

Throughout this time, in the presence of the background noise in my head, I had been actively searching for answers and was trying hard to find ways to circumvent my symptoms or devise strategies to live with the symptoms. I realized that my focus was life! The core motivation for my searches and struggles was because I wanted to continue living. I realized that, yet again, I had to make a conscious decision to live.

I'm pretty sure that many of the episodes of my more recent symptoms could have been fear induced, because the symptoms have receded significantly since the consciousness of living became apparent to me. Dr. Joe Dispenza's book, *You Are the Placebo: Making Your Mind Matter* suggests that we really are the placebos we need. A belief in life and a future will manifest itself in reality.

The truth about cancer is that there *are* stories that defy science and I believe with all my heart you can be one of those stories as well. This is one place that the cliché, "If I can do it, you can do it" really applies. If you paid attention to the data in the introduction, you will have noticed that survivors are in the majority and you are statistically more likely to live than to die with a cancer diagnosis.

Cancer makes us feel like we have to rely on doctors to find a cure. The result is that we relinquish our power and responsibility for our own healing to someone else. Our western medical model has taught us that we are not as knowledgeable as our doctors. They are esteemed and put on the highest pedestals in society. We can become so reliant on them that we do not trust our opinions and ourselves regarding our approach to healing from cancer. After all, medical science has spent billions on research to understand this disease. Surely we know less about this disease than they do. No we don't. We know a whole lot more about ourselves than they do, so we are well equipped to find our cures.

Here is the challenge to that thinking: Medical practitioners have not been educated in the science of life. Their craft is about trying to understand disease and to cure it. Through this lens, their focus has to be on the disease, not you, necessarily. When you start asking doctors questions that are important to you, you will hear answers about their experience with this disease, which, according to the current track record, is not that great. I have yet to hear of doctors who loudly proclaim that they can cure a cancer patient. They will carefully answer your question, "Can you cure me?" or "Will this cure me?" with a convoluted way of saying, "I cannot make that claim." They know little about each of us; the people who have renegade cells behaving badly inside of us. Typically, doctors have known us only for a few hours when we have these discussions, and all they have read are MRI test and scan results. They have knowledge about the statistical odds and research evidence, based on studying others with this disease, not us as individuals.

How can they possibly know what we have learned about life and living from our own perspectives? How do they know our strengths, beliefs and how we face a challenge? They don't! And very few of them ask the questions to find that out about us. Instead, they go into attack or defense mode completely focused on fighting cancer cells. They know about the tools they have to kill cells in the human body. They have the skill to excise a tumor and patch up the incision. They know nothing about how we fight or defend ourselves and many times we have not consciously thought about these things either.

I have great respect for the great doctors who I have encountered. They are well educated, knowledgeable and many are wise. You will encounter skilled physicians, too. Still, they cannot know enough about you for them to help you to be fully healed. It is up to you to take the lead, to teach them about your perspectives so that together you can make a real difference to your outcomes.

Start thinking about yourself as head of the team and that, together, you are setting out to succeed at the biggest goal of your life. In order to succeed you have to reevaluate your stance about wanting to live and proclaim it consciously. Now you can start uncovering your collective knowledge and mobilizing your team, your body, mind and spirit into being an effective healing machine. If you have doubts about your ability to do this, think about this: Have you ever broken a bone? If you have, all the doctor did was put your limb in a cast to immobilize it. No magical healing powers, no medications were prescribed to heal the bone. You did that. Your body is a miraculous healing machine. It knows how to heal broken bones, for heaven's sake! It fights infection and cancer every day, too, without degrees and research to back itself up. It just does it.

That is the power you can learn to use in this fight. Your doctor can't do that for you.

Don't let your doubts bully you into thinking that you are powerless to beat cancer and that someone else has all the answers. You have enough self-knowledge to have an opinion; many opinions about life and living. Use those to kick the healing knowledge inside your body into action and learn all you can from outside sources of how best to address the cancer. You are not a victim whose only option is to be pushed into making rash decisions that might go against your deep inner convictions. Pause and think about those convictions, your strength and your need for resources to mobilize the best team to help you through this. You might want to write this conviction in your journal to use later when you need some convincing again.

What has evolved with the development of Western medicine is a reliance purely on the skills and knowledge of the medical practitioner or medical science as a whole. We have relinquished the power over our health and healing to outside entities. It is time for us to work together as a real team and to share the responsibility.

It doesn't matter if the outside entity to which you assign power over your healing comes from a medical, nutritional or alternative healing background. The key is, that in order to live again after being diagnosed with cancer, you have to recognize your personal responsibility to taking charge of your healing; taking charge of life. You can and should be the head of the healing team, taking charge of your health approaches and finding your cure from a deeply personal perspective that matches your beliefs, temperament and tendencies.

If you want to fight, then assume the stance of a fighter with your army alongside you. If you prefer to embrace a less aggressive approach and want to enhance your health, then embrace the role of healer with your advisors there to support you. If you have not yet assembled the perfect team or approach, go for a second or third opinion. Seek information and alternatives and assemble the best team possible to give you the support and tools to outlive this cancer. There is no rush. If you feel that you have to move quickly, do so. But do so thoughtfully and strategically to gather more information so you can build your team and create your cure. It took me three months to assemble my strategy and my team of healers when I was diagnosed with a tumor that engulfed my breast and caused liver and lung metastases. During that time, I had no real clue as to what I was going to do to beat the cancer. All I knew is what I *wouldn't do* and that was chemotherapy or have a radical mastectomy.

Two different teams of oncologists had two different opinions about the surgery; I latched onto the one that felt right to me. I didn't think I should lop off the offending boob. My reasoning was that it would leave me trying to recover from surgery while still having the tumors in my left lung and liver. Those were far scarier to me than the origin of the disease. It was almost like I had accepted that I had a bad boob, but that I needed to focus my attention on the more life-giving organs in my body. That, at that time, was the first life-giving decision that I made. My family and people around me thought that I was crazy, but they accepted my decision a lot easier than the surgeon who proclaimed, "You *will* have a radical mastectomy on Tuesday."

I was in Northern Indiana when this diagnosis had been made and, luckily for me, the executive director of the clinic I was working in gave me a referral to a surgeon who was a colleague and friend at the Rush Cancer Institute in Chicago. I made the appointment to go to Rush on Wednesday, the day after the local surgeon wanted me to have a radical mastectomy. When the local surgeon became frustrated with me about not agreeing to make the appointment for the mastectomy, he and the oncologist who was on the panel proved that they were not listening to me and that their decision was final. The oncologist chimed in that I would wake up from surgery with the first intravenous dose of chemo already being delivered and that I would lose all my hair as a result of the chemo he would be prescribing. My stubborn answer, for the third time was, "No I won't," to which the oncologist became visibly angry with me and stated, "I have been doing this for over 30 years and every patient I have given this chemo to has lost their hair!" My reply was simply, "I understand, that, doctor, but I will never be a patient of yours so I will not lose my hair." At this point he stormed out. The surgeon gave it one more try, emboldened by his colleague's stern behavior and he wanted to know what on earth I thought was more important than having the mastectomy and starting chemo. My simple reply was, "Having a second opinion."

He calmed down a little when he heard that who I had an appointment with was his mentor and surgical idol and said, "Please come back and let me know what he says. I think he will either tell you that I am the most brilliant surgeon or the biggest fool." I had the courage to return to his office a week later to tell him that, based on the reason his mentor gave for not performing any surgery, the latter applied. Years later, when my healer and amazing oncologist looked back on that decision, he told me that it would not have been possible to remove the whole breast tumor in those early days of the disease. The surgeon would have cut through the tumor, which by its nature, would never have healed, as normal tissue would have. That stubborn decision saved my life. At the time, though, that decision still left me with no clue about what to do about the metastases. I had stood my ground about not having chemo again, but did accept a hormone-blocking pill instead. The doctors told me that I was not aggressively killing the cancer and doubted that what I was allowing them to do enough. I even had an encounter with a nurse who proclaimed with authority that, "We know that patients with liver or lung cancer do not survive." I was shocked and infuriated, so I marched into her office and told her that she had no right to declare me as a candidate for death and that I would prove her wrong. I could have lost my job over that, but the anger it fueled was good for me; it helped me survive so I would keep my word and indeed prove her wrong. She told me later that I had given her one of her life lessons.

Three months into searching for other ways to fight cancer effectively, I met two amazing healers, one a dedicated cancer nutritionist and the other, who I fondly refer to as my wholeness coach. The truth, though, was that at this time the medication was not working, and the changes in my diet and lifestyle had not had time to have an impact. A new tumor appeared in my lung and one in my liver had increased in size. This irked the oncologist to a point that she actively ignored me, telling me at my last appointment with her (before I fired her, that is), that she forgot that I was in the examination room for almost two hours because she was dealing with a very serious obstacle in her research. I took that as meaning that her research was far more important than me, so I walked out, and cancelled any future appointments. I needed an ally in my quest for living, not a devoted researcher.

My primary physician helped me find the third person in my healing team, a local oncologist in Indiana, who understood that each person has a unique way of living with cancer. Since he had not studied the alternative approaches I was taking, he could not tell me if they would work, but what he did was endorse and support my endeavors. He liked that I was taking a holistic approach with several angles to support my body to be efficient and to rid me of cancer. His contribution was to tell me that breast cancer was no longer seen by him as a life-threatening disease; only a chronic one similar to diabetes. Like with diabetes, his belief was that if you manage the disease, people with cancer can have a long life. He discussed the many tools that he had, other than chemo, and helped me to decide on a more targeted hormone-blocking injection that was given once a month. The most important thing that this amazing healer and oncologist did during my first appointment was to give me a hug. He was a mensch – a real human being who saw me as a real human being. He gave me the physical and mental affirmation that we were in this together and that we could succeed if we worked together. A year later this special oncologist declared that all my scans showed no evidence of tumors in my liver or lung.

I had worked hard at listening, learning and embracing approaches that felt right for me, and that I could do diligently with the belief that it all would work to overcome the cancer and that I would live. It did! You can too! I know that in your head are a lot of objections, "yes, buts" that take over. So let's take a moment and address all of your doubts and fears. You may feel that you don't have enough knowledge about all the options. You may feel that you are not as courageous or adventurous as I was. But you might be thinking that I am different and special.

No, I'm not any different from you. I was scared out of my wits!!! Both times! The difference is that the first time I had zero knowledge and zero alternatives. I felt like a feather in the wind. I was told to go for this test, so I did. I was told I would have that needle stuck into me, so I did. I was told to make an appointment to see this specialist, so I did. I was told what chemo I would have and how it would be dosed for six months immediately followed by daily radiation for six weeks, and I did. I was asked hundreds of questions and filled out pages of questionnaires about family histories and all that emerged was a sinking realization that I was surrounded by people on both sides of my family who had died of cancer. I remember saying out loud over and over when walking to radiation departments, imaging departments for every body part, "I am not a cancer patient!" The soft, sympathetic smiles that humored me with that thought tried to tell me that I *was, in fact, with proof, a cancer patient.*

In the end, I had nothing, except a sinking realization that the signs surrounding me were right. I was a cancer patient.

An interesting thing happened on the first Friday after my first diagnosis and after a whole week of tests and scans, doctor's appointments and needle sticks. I had my results appointment with the surgeon who I was told would make the first decision about my treatment protocols. In the midst of him relating back to me all the results and the indications from my family history, I remembered my great aunt Suzie, who had been diagnosed with breast cancer as a young woman and again when she was 80. I blurted out defiantly, "And she lived to the ripe old age of 92 and died of natural causes. I'm going to be just like her!" That was my first moment of hope and clarity. Everything else pointed to a miserable truth, but that realization was powerful enough to get me through. I had found one little beacon of hope and was determined to hold onto it for dear life. After all, I had five young daughters, the youngest of whom was about to turn one year old. I could not die and leave them to grow up without me. You might not have a great aunt Suzie, or five daughters to live for, but you can make the decision to outlive cancer.

Pause a moment, think about your reason to live. Write it down, etch it into your heart and mind and your spirit will start to see that there is a way you *can* and will do this! Stand up to all the objections in your head and say, even if it is with a weak voice initially, *I will outlive cancer!* Say it again: ***I will outlive cancer.*** Now use that statement every day as a positive affirmation every hour. Set an alarm in your phone and read it out loud if you can. Your brain needs something to help it believe in and to sort out what it needs to be doing internally to mobilize healing. Give it that belief in itself, even when you haven't arrived at being fully convinced yourself yet.

Congratulations! You have started your empowering journey. You *will* outlive cancer! All my reading, listening to audios, going to seminars in my search to understand cancer, helped me figure out how to overcome it and live life again. I have read books that taught me about the mind-body connection, about visualization, guided imagery, diet, breathing and meditation. Seminars and workshops helped me understand different perspectives, gather practices and learn techniques that I have been able to pass on to others to help in their cures as well. Something I learned is that medical science has not figured out what the essence of life is. Each one of us has it within us. Each of us defines and experiences it differently. Some find it in their faith practices, some in nature. Now is a good time for you to get in touch with that life inside you. What does it mean to you to be alive? Write your answer down. That revelation or meaning that you give life is the secret of outliving cancer. Don't be silly and think you don't need anything else. You do need other things for your body, but for now, be alive and make that commitment to yourself to *live*. That is what I call *Living Life Loudly*. It is about embracing the life within you, around you and through every sense in your body. It is about experiencing life with a fresh appreciation of what you have, through smelling life with all its ugly smells as well as the fragrant ones; sensing it through your eyes and skin, through your ears and tongue. It is like falling in love with your life because you have life. Your brain will embrace the endorphins and other hormones that you release with this living life loudly and get to work to make your body more efficient. Medicine cannot give you that. This will be the new way you look at your solutions and find your cure. My motto, stolen from the Jewish toast, is: "L'Chaim!" It means "To Life!" Join me in celebrating yours.

In this chapter I introduced you to the idea that you have a life to live, even if you have been diagnosed with cancer. Cancer did not give you a reason for your life before your diagnosis and it shouldn't define your life now. Finding your passion and reason for living will help you find how you are going to approach the rest of your life. Life is a celebration when it has meaning. Cancer may have temporary control over the emotions attached to life, but cannot rob us of the way we choose to live our lives. Doing the purpose exercise is a way to clarify our "why," and next, I will show you ways to figure out the "how."

Now let's get to work.

Chapter 2

THE FOUR PILLARS OF HEALING

We are ready to start working on the task of figuring out what the best approaches are for you to deal with the cancer in your life. I have divided these into four categories which I think are pillars of healing. Sorting approaches into these four categories will help reduce the overwhelm and give you a place to start.

The most common thread I hear from newly diagnosed cancer patients is being overwhelmed. Cancer overwhelms us with emotion and we are immediately thrust into an overload of information. The barrage of information about tests, treatment options and strategies are usually presented with little help on how to process the information or deal with the emotions. Without a frame of reference of how to break everything down and to simplify it, we are left feeling helpless, sad and afraid. We have no clue where to begin and are unable to make informed decisions crucial in our recovery and healing. This is not a good place to start fighting cancer.

A good place to start is to sit down with a piece of paper and pen and create a mind map by writing down what you do know so far. This helps to start the process of organizing your thoughts about what you are facing, how your belief system helps you make sense of the diagnosis and what is being offered to you as possible approaches for a cure.

Ask yourself, "What do I already know?" Write down all your thoughts, as haphazardly as they come. You can make sense of them once you stop writing.

The second question to answer is, "What do I want to find out and know about my cancer?" Think about questions you have about your options, what options have you heard about and want to explore to learn more about. Write all these down; they will help you search for answers more clearly. A third question you might want to ask is, "What do I *not* know about this cancer and its treatment?" This might lead you to explore holistic alternatives, concepts like mind-body approaches and other resources that you had not considered. It may lead you to find out about ways to deal with your appearance before you start chemo for example. Write these thoughts down as well.

Now you can sort through the answers, the new questions and the gaps in your knowledge that you want to fill. Write the thoughts and ideas that crystalize from this exercise into your journal. It will help you know where you can make a start. Most treatment centers try to give you lots of alternatives, but too much information coming at you while still trying to process the diagnosis can have the reverse effect of immobilizing you with overwhelm.

The easiest way that I have found to deal with this is to tackle questions about cancer using the four pillars of healing.

For me, these are:
1. Mind
2. Body
3. Spirit
4. Support

I have divided this book into these four sections for that reason. If you haven't already, now would be a good time to start a journal to capture the organized thoughts from your mind maps previously done and as a companion for capturing the thoughts and feelings as you read this book, and to complete the writing and drawing assignments I suggest later.

SECTION 1

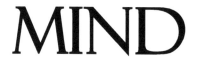

MIND

Chapter 3

EMOTIONS

───────────~───────────

Emotions are what drive our thoughts in relation to cancer. If we allow the emotions to take over and rule us, cancer becomes a very hard thing to overcome. If we recognize, identify, name and face the emotions, we have a better chance of using our minds to fight cancer. When diagnosed with cancer, our minds have just been forced to alter everything we believe about our lives. Life, how long we imagined we would live, our vitality and our longevity are all thrown into turmoil with one little sentence – you have cancer. It is mind numbing.

The media, our community experiences, the stories that we remember about others with cancer, take our minds to dark places of despair. Places where our minds dwell on what can go wrong and that things have already gone wrong, rather than going to places of joy and hope.

Typically joy and hope don't enter our minds and people around us who try to get us to be hopeful and to look on the bright side are thought of as being out of touch with what we have to deal with. I know for me, in the beginning I wanted to scream out aloud at these people who had no idea what I was going through and to shut up and leave me alone rather than to try to fill my mind with positive platitudes. My most fierce thoughts were towards people in the medical profession who spoke down to me like I had somehow become incapable of understanding the English language and that they had to speak slower and softer to me with an upward inflection at the end of every sentence, like you would speak to a child. Cancer does not change who we are, not our brains, not our minds and not our maturity.

The solution for regaining your control over this disease and over your integrity is to gain control of your mind. Here are some ideas that might help with that.

Making sense of the turmoil is important. Dr. Bernie Siegel, author of *Love, Medicine and Miracles,* one of the first books to offer me some hope and real strategies to deal with my diagnosis, suggested to all his new cancer patients to draw a picture of their cancer, their treatment and their cure. I suggest that you take a moment to draw your own picture of you, the cancer and the cure.

It is important to process what the diagnosis means to you. If you don't draw, create a mind map with the word **cancer** in the center of the page and capture all your thoughts relating to the word, linking like spokes of a wheel. Words like fear, grief, sadness and helplessness will reveal your frame of thought. Keep writing until you cannot come up with any more thoughts about cancer. Do the same with the word **treatment** and, lastly, write the word **cure** on a page and capture all your thoughts about that.

This exercise will reveal to you your overall mindset about cancer. Now you have to make a choice: Do you approve of living with this mindset or not? What will you embrace as part of your mindset in fighting cancer and what do you want to change? This might lead to a new drawing or page of insights. You are now ready to embark on strategies to deal with the mental aspect of fighting cancer.

There are no right or wrong thoughts and emotions. They are just thoughts and emotions. Dr. Siegel suggests that if you think a thought is corrosive and damaging to your overall well-being, write all you can about this thought on paper. It can take the form of a letter or just your most detailed descriptions about these thoughts and the fears they elicit. Acknowledge that they are now outside your body, on the paper, where they no longer can do you any harm, then destroy the piece of paper, symbolically destroying the power these thoughts have over you. I remember my pen ripping through the paper as I did this exercise the first time. I was so angry and resentful that I destroyed the page before I was supposed to.

We are told to be positive or to avoid negative thoughts when we have to fight cancer. Well, that may be true, but we aren't given any ideas on how to block the negative thoughts or what to do with them. You can start with writing what you consider to be the negative emotions down on paper, they are now outside your body. Now symbolically destroy the feelings by destroying the paper you wrote them on. It is OK to have evidence of a ripped out page that reminds you that you successfully got rid of those emotions. It is OK if you have to do this exercise more than once. Strong emotions have a habit of returning. Now you know how to deal with them. I know this sounds overly simplistic. But when I learned about this tool, it was all I had and it helped. Nothing else was helping.

I will go through a list of thoughts and emotions that commonly accompany the diagnosis of cancer with some suggestions of how to use or alter the power and energy these emotions evoke. I identify five key emotions as being: sad, mad, bad, scared and glad. If you give the cerebral cortex something to do with emotion, like give it a name, it can help you cope with the emotion. If you don't actually say what the emotion is, then you can easily be held hostage to the emotion and get trapped there and not move forward.

Let's name each emotion.

Sad

The first emotion that seems to be the big problem with being given a diagnosis of cancer is sadness, sometimes thought of as depression. It's not really depression it's grief. Have you thought of that? There's no pill that can fix grief, emptiness or sadness. If it's called depression then psychologists, psychiatrists and doctors often just want to give us a pill and make it go away. That is not going to help. It's not going to take the cancer away. It's not going to take the sadness away. Acknowledge the sadness and sit with it for a while. Give it a name. Say out aloud something like: "The problem is that I'm feeling sad or numb. The problem is that I'm feeling a sense of loss or grief." Sadness can be experienced as feeling numb or emotionless, in a trance or in a stunned silence. Once you acknowledge the emotion, that allows you the space to either grieve it, feel it or process it. The cerebral cortex now has something to do with the emotion. Your thoughts will start doing their job of comprehending sadness and its meaning in your situation and will ultimately reveal what can be done about it. You can consciously ask sadness what it is trying to say to you. Write down the thoughts that come to you about your sadness.

What can you do about sadness? Sadness is often as a result of a sense of loss. I know for me, the sense of loss was that I would no longer be able to do what I wanted to do. I was forced to think I no longer could dream about the life that I thought I had ahead of me. I was no longer able to see a future with grown-up daughters and in general, see my future. There were things that I had taken for granted that would be in my future like the possibility of travel. Sadness robbed me of my sense of myself in the future. I saw nothing. I had to understand that this sense of loss was what I needed to grieve. You don't suddenly just think, "Oh, well. Now I've got cancer and these things might not happen in my life." There is a primitive part of our brain that takes over this emotion and can exaggerate it till it is totally out of control. You have to recognize it and do something about it. Just acknowledging sadness, that it's not depression, that it is, in fact, a sense of grief and loss can help you do something about it.

You can allow yourself a process or create a process. Some people like to write and writing it down, journaling about those emotions, journaling about that sadness, the loss is very healthy. Some people paint or play the piano, or an instrument, listen to music or plain and simple sit down and cry.

I have a friend who went through a series of losses. She hadn't grieved the loss of her mother, she hadn't grieved the loss of her marriage, or the loss of her country. Over time she was overwhelmed by grief and sadness. Talking through it with her counselor, what she found helpful was to set an alarm clock for an hour and say, "Okay, now I'm going to sit here and cry." She would cry her heart out, but when the alarm went off she would stop crying and say, "That's it. You've done your crying for today. Now you've got other things to do," and she would move on. After some time she needed the alarm clock less and less, and she needed those moments of crying every day less and less.

If you recognize that cancer steers you into this sense of loss and grief, and you can identify what it is that you're grieving and what you want to do about it, it restores your power. Not completely, but it gives you back enough power so you can be more assertive and be more in charge.

The second time that I was diagnosed with cancer I felt that I'd had the privilege of experiencing cancer once before and had been successful in overcoming it. I believed that, for the most part, my children's experience of the first cancer was that they had not been burdened by it or by what I was going through. Some of them were too little. However, they did remember the better moments, times when we were able to laugh at cancer. So when I brought up the fact that it had been a good learning experience for what we were facing the second time, they seemed to embrace that mindset and hold on to the good parts of the experience to color the new cancer experience.

Just after I was diagnosed the second time, while I was waiting for the panel discussion to outline test findings and treatment options, a young man came up to me, and called me by my first name. I didn't know him from Adam. Coming from a rigid South African background, I was a bit offended by a stranger not addressing me more formally. He introduced himself as the psychology intern who was going to "take care of my depression." I took even more offense to being told that I was depressed.

The poor guy had started off on the wrong foot and proceeded to step deeper into a hole. He had already labeled me as having depression before even speaking to me. I knew that I didn't have depression, so I challenged him. I asked him, "Where did you get that idea, that I had depression, or I was suffering from depression?" He said, "Because of your diagnosis." I said, "My diagnosis is not me and because I have a diagnosis of cancer, does that mean that I get labeled as being cancerous and depressive?" He was embarrassed. I continued without much thought for his discomfort and said, "The other thing is, professionals don't talk about this here in a public waiting room." He hurried me into a private office.

I said to him, "What I'm experiencing is a sense of loss, a sense of loss of vitality and of the possibility of my future. I sense the loss of my future and question if I will be able to do my job. That's not depression, that's pretty healthy, normal grieving, I am processing my potential losses. Your labeling it as depression is counter-productive. It's not helping me process my current situation. I don't want to overcome this emotion, I want to process this emotion and if you haven't got anything to help me do that with, then this meeting's over."

Because I was such a bitch he was apologetic and he said, "I just failed Psychology 101; I should have asked and listened to you to find out what you are experiencing and how you were experiencing it, rather than labeling." As a result, he became a pretty good resource for me. He gave me books about grief and audios that helped me process grief through activities and guided imagery; all things that were really useful to me. The point here is that you must identify the sadness, recognize it and label it. Then understand what it is that you want from the people around you in order to process the sadness. When you take the diagnostic labeling out of your sadness and talk about what's going on inside, you really can start processing and understanding what this disease is doing to you and what it means in your life. You can't take the fear, the guilt and the sting out of this experience, but you can diminish it. You're not supposed to eradicate these negative thoughts and feelings. You have to understand them for what they are.

At the beginning of this chapter, you may have thought, "I have to get into a positive frame of mind or mindset." No. Not necessarily. The point about having emotions is that all emotions are neutral. Some emotions seem to be positive, others negative and there is an ebb and flow between emotions. We do not have to be in the positive scale of emotion and live our lives there. It would really be a flat world if we did that. In addition, that expectation puts way too much pressure on us to be or feel what we are not. It's healthy to have the emotions that we call negative emotions, like sadness. Dwelling in the emotion for months or years is what causes the problem.

Keep practicing, recognizing and processing. Writing it down, understanding it and calling it what it is. Then, taking it along with you for the journey, because it really is a discovery journey.

Mad

Let's move on to the second emotion, mad - anger. Anger can take the form of frustration, feeling trapped and feeling stuck with this diagnosis. What has happened to your health was not your choice! It happened to you, was done to you, forced upon you and you might be justified in being angry. You might want to lash out and fight. I know that initially, whenever things didn't go according to my plan, or to my thinking of how it should go, I would lash out. I could be the royal bitch and I think I turned well-meaning people away because of my lashing out. The anger was not a bad thing. It was my behavior that was bad. The truth about anger is that it often masks being afraid.

What you need to do with anger is recognize that it's present and that it's a healthy way of processing cancer. I like to say, "You have to shake the shit off your shoe." You've got to get rid of the sadness, yes. Then deal with the anger, which you may be directing at yourself and at your body. What are you angry about? Let's process this. Ask your mind to help you and write down what you hear.

A healthy way to start is to think about what triggers the anger. Is it the cancer or is it the anger of what the cancer is doing to you? Who is cancer doing something to other than yourself? Cancer affects a lot of people around us. Are you angry that your children might not see you grow to a ripe, old age? Are you angry that you might miss out on their experiences and watch them grow and have experiences you would like for them? Dig deep and look at what the anger really means and then recognize what triggers the anger.

People who triggered anger in me when I was fighting cancer were the ones who were overly soft spoken and came at me with this powder puff of feeling sorry for me. They were so phony; it made me want to scream with anger. You've got to recognize what triggers that anger and then see what physical responses you have. I found that my back would go straight or my jaw would clench. My hands would make fists and I would go into an aggressive stance with a stern facial expression. If you can recognize your physical response to the anger, you can probably block the lashing out that might follow. It takes practice. Becoming a saint is not what I suggest; just don't let the anger get in the way of your healing support system by damaging relationships that matter. Recognize the trigger. Recognize the changes in your body. Does your blood pressure go up? Do you get red in the face? Do you leap up and want to do something physical? The point here is not to suppress it. Don't allow it to take control of you and result in your becoming an angry person. You might also want to look at what fears are triggering the anger. Make the effort to see what choices you have to shift this anger.

Newton's second law of energy states that energy is never lost or found; it is only transferred. Anger is energy and can be transferred but we have to learn to transfer anger satisfactorily, without transferring it inwards where it potentially can do you a lot of harm. Listen to the language you use to describe what anger does to you. I used to get so angry about things that I would say, "It's eating me up inside." And then, guess what? I was diagnosed with cancer. It is vital to transfer anger by finding practices that would satisfactorily transfer the energy into something productive. Transferring the energy into vigorous physical activity like a sport, walking, running or even scrubbing a floor are healthy examples.

The first time I was diagnosed with cancer I was 40. The second time I was diagnosed was just after I had turned 54. I had become fat and lazy and with tumors in my lung it had become physically challenging to start moving. I knew that exercise was a way to beat cancer. I forced myself to start walking as vigorously and with as much determination as I could. This was a way that I could process the anger as well as giving me something positive to channel the anger through. At first, I was able to reach the driveway of the house two doors down. I started a mantra that helped me hold onto the reason for walking. It went like this, "I'm going to walk this cancer right out of my life." I continued to stomp my way around the neighborhood with this mantra firmly fixed in my mind. Walking the emotion off made me feel that I was making a physical difference to my body's functioning. Before I left Indiana, I was able to walk three miles briskly. It helped to have one of my neighbors, an athlete, come along and challenge me to go just a little further with every walk. When I turned 60 I ran my very first mile ever!

I had learned that I enjoyed being physically competitive. I loved going to the gym. I loved running. I loved riding my bike. I would push myself really hard. It was an effective way for me to dissipate my aggressions.

I was 64 and very fit at the time of my third diagnosis. Because the cancer affected my cardiac function I couldn't move without chest pain and shortness of breath. I couldn't push my body. I couldn't dissipate that anger or transfer it the same way anymore. I had to find a new way to challenge my body.

I tried Tai Chi but didn't allow it to benefit me. I was too judgmental about the precision and called it slow. I had a bad attitude towards yoga too, saying that it would bore me because it wasn't ballistic, fast or resistive enough for me.

I was wrong. I was introduced to yoga when my back had gone into spasm; another sign of how angry I was with the world. I had to go for physical therapy. My physical therapist was a movement specialist and yoga instructor. He had me doing lots of stretching. While I was doing these stretches, I could feel my body start to release. I could also feel when my body stopped wanting to release and that was a challenge. Every time I would pull my face, he would say, "Okay, well that's tough, how about if you just breathe and hold that stretch for a minute and see what happens? See if your body will let it go."

Lo and behold, it did! Of course, I wasn't "doing yoga" at that stage, I was stretching. The home program sheet my therapist gave me was labeled "stretches" but he kept encouraging me to join a yoga class. Finally, when I went to one of his yoga classes, I discovered that all the "stretches" I had been doing for restoring my body to its normal function were part of yoga. My judgment had been that yoga was boring and was for wimps. I had quite a big surprise ahead of me, because by the end of that first yoga class I was sweating, I was sore and I almost felt defeated, but mostly challenged by how difficult yoga was. But you know what? I wasn't angry any more. I felt pretty good about the accomplishment of twisting my body and holding poses in spite of them being well beyond my physical flexibility!

I lay on the mat afterwards and got the giggles because I had seen that I could challenge my body in a completely different way without having to do a hard cardio workout. I could transfer my angry energy without having to be a badass.

Here is a challenge for you: Find something physical that challenges you, absorbs your attention and helps you to dissipate the anger. It could even be something like playing the piano. When I was a kid, I use to play the piano when I was angry. I would start out banging the keys. My mother would yell at me, "Stop banging the keys!" I was angry, so I would continue to bang the keys. After a while, that key banging became less satisfying; it no longer sounded good, the energy had shifted and I found myself playing something that was loud and fast initially, and eventually playing something that was soft and beautiful. The energy would shift and with it the anger did too.

Explore things that help you transfer your anger. It could be doing push-ups against the kitchen sink or digging in the garden. It could be walking as vigorously as you can to the neighbor's driveway. Do anything, but do move. Find something to help you shift that energy away from the emotion you don't like and the behavior you don't like to something that is satisfying. It is possible. All you have to do is sit and think about it then commit to it.

Writing is another strategy that can help to shift emotion. I learned this from Dr. Bernie Siegel in his book, *Love, Medicine and Miracles*. Write down your anger. I used to write so hard that I would tear the paper as my pen ripped through what I was angry about. Dr. Siegel suggests that once written, the anger is outside of you; now destroy the anger symbolically by tearing the paper up, burning it, crumpling it up or shredding it. So satisfying! Dr. Siegel adds, "If you harbor the anger inside you, it will do physical harm." So, you take it out of you, put it on a piece of paper that you can destroy once you have written all the venom onto the page. As a result, it becomes an emotion that is outside of you and can no longer turn into cancer.

Bad

Having so-called negative emotions like anger and sadness can lead to feeling bad about having those emotions and for acting out your emotions in some cases. Guilt can be related to your thoughts that you won't be there for people who you love, guilty that you've been angry or that you've been withdrawn. You could be feeling guilty that you're sick or guilty that you puked on the neighbor's daffodils during your chemo. Again, you can't magically get rid of the guilt by saying, "Well, I shouldn't be feeling guilty." You have to learn and understand the guilt to process it. The problem with guilt is that you really are judging yourself. When you judge yourself, it can get so bad that it turns into self-loathing, especially when you have cancer. That self-loathing can trap you and be like a ball and chain around your ankle.

Freedom comes from choosing to learn and understand, rather than judge. I learned this from Marilee Adams, Ph.D., a professor of psychology and learning. Something she talks and writes about, is that life takes you along a pathway of choices. The pathway is often unfamiliar and your choices are either to take the learner pathway or the judging pathway. When you choose not to judge, you open yourself to learning. If you judge, no learning can happen and you eventually start judging yourself for being stuck with the consequences of the judgment. You have the choice to switch to learning at any time during the journey. That is when we start to learn real life lessons.

Think of a topic that you want to learn about. If I said to you, "Well that's the dumbest thing, why do you want to learn about that?" I'm judging you. What might happen to you? You either defend your desire to learn or you might start judging yourself. When you fall into the trap of judging, it eventually leads you to think, "Well, maybe it *is* a dumb idea to learn about this topic."

Dr. Adams says that at any point that you find yourself falling into that judgment path, that you can actually turn around and start to learn. Ask yourself this simple question: "Do I choose to learn and understand what's happening right now?" Dr. Adams has a choice map, which you can download for free at her, website: www.inquiryinstitute.com. Print it and pin it up in front of you to help you be reminded that there is always something you can learn in every situation. Whatever you blame yourself for, cancer is not your fault. You might not think that cancer causes you to blame yourself, but the more you learn about what causes cancer and about your lifestyles, you can easily start blaming yourself for not eating the right foods or consuming too much sugar or for smoking or not exercising enough. Those are all judgments and they result in you feeling guilty.

Consciously start looking at what you judge yourself for, then apply the first step of healing: forgive yourself. The second step to changing the bad feeling is to ask what it is you need to learn in order to change the situation. Ask yourself that question and let it sit there for a bit. Write down what you learn. The third step is to choose to follow that learning path. Carrying out these three steps will help process guilt without sucking you into the vortex of self-loathing and hate for being the cancer patient, for being a bad cancer patient, for getting cancer in the first place, for allowing your immune system to break down – blah, blah, blah. Choose to learn and see what it is you can change. Your life will benefit from it.

Scared

The fourth emotion we face as cancer patients is being scared. You have cancer and that is scary, I understand, but you have to ask: what is that fear? You're probably thinking, "Hell yeah, I'm scared, what is she thinking and where has she been?" The problem with being scared or fearful is not facing the fear and not facing what might happen if you stay scared. If you wrap yourself up in fear and hide, you will never beat cancer. You have to recognize that you are scared, probably scared witless, and then analyze it so that you can understand it.

Ask yourself what are you afraid of? How does this fear manifest? What does this fear tell you the outcome of your cancer is going to be? How do you experience the fear? It is important to look at the fear and to question fear. This helps you get out of fear and help you discover what you need to cure the cancer. Remember anger? Anger is often the guise for fear.

Fear is a good thing because it mobilizes you. If it doesn't, then you're going to be that scared person with your head under the pillow curled up, trying to escape. That's not a way to beat cancer. When you are scared, enlist someone to support you through the scary times. Having someone next to you in a scary movie helps you get through the horrific parts. It is the same with cancer. Support makes this journey easier. If you do not have close family and friends, find a support group. You might be surprised and find a cure together.

Glad

The fifth emotion is gladness or happiness. You might think, "Okay, I don't really know what I'm supposed to do to be happy about regarding cancer." Cancer robs of you of feeling glad or of any shade of happiness. That's the truth. You're living it right now. It sucks the happiness and the joy out of the lives of the people around you, too, initially. This does change, however, when you do something to seek happiness and laughter actively. How? You might ask, especially after I've suggested you dwell in the sadness for a while so you can understand it. I've told you to look at your anger so you can figure it out and use the energy to move yourself physically. I've told you to look at where you feel guilty and feel bad about the failure of your body to thrive. If paying so much attention to the negative emotions, how on earth are you supposed to feel glad?

One of the ways to do it is to fake it until you make it. The hospice in Johannesburg, where a friend worked, had a happiness activity every day. To my mind, people in a hospice were either in pretty bad shape or were dying. I thought the happiness activity was the most asinine thing that I had ever heard of! Why were they forcing people who were dying to be happy? The physiology of laughter, whether the laughter is genuine or forced, is that laughter releases endorphins in the brain. Endorphins have the power to reduce pain, lift the mood and kick your immune system into being healthy and efficient. Isn't that what you want your body to do so you can fight cancer? Pretty smart, those hospice workers who helped people laugh.

When I decided that I was going to do all that I could to kick every cell in my body into high gear to recognize bad cells and work towards a living goal, I knew that I had to lighten up. I sent my husband out to go and buy me the box set of the Marx Brothers movies. I knew that even when I was in a bad mood, eventually the Marx Brothers would elicit at least one laugh out of me. Maybe sometimes it wasn't a laugh; it was a little squeaky smile. But it worked. My goal of living life without cancer or the fear of it coming back wasn't always easy and laughter was one of those things that eventually made a difference to my mindset.

I started loosening up and stopped judging the stupid things that I laughed at or the stupidity in comedies. My father didn't have much of a sense of humor. My mother loved comedy, so we often went to watch British comedy shows. I could hear my father mutter under his breath, and sometimes not so softly, "This is so stupid. This British humor is stupid. I can't relate to it." I had adopted the same narrow view, so slapstick would get on my nerves and I would become annoyed by it. Consciously wanting to fight cancer changed that and I learned to choose to relax, not judge and to start laughing at stupid things.

You've got to find the humor that works for you. I have found, because I'm South African, I relate to Trevor Noah.

When I'm feeling angry or just downright sad, I force myself to go downstairs and watch an episode of Trevor Noah's "*Today Show*." Somehow his foolishness and humor can make me laugh, making me feel better. The purpose of court jesters was to make the king to feel happy and good about all the bad things in royal life. Cancer is the bad thing happening in your life. Get rid of that cancer with laughter. Find something or someone that makes you laugh. You might not see it right now, but it is a great way to work on a cure.

When I was first diagnosed, a woman called Eileen came to visit me. I only knew Eileen by her reputation as an auspicious figure in our church – she was an English teacher and school principal. I'm a little intimidated by people like that because I never think my language, accent or diction are good enough. This beautifully spoken, intimidating person came knocking on my front door after I was diagnosed with cancer. It was during a pretty dark time for me. After my surgery I felt that people were diminishing me. They treated me as though I wasn't capable of getting up out of bed to get a drink or make myself something to eat. I hated it. I hated it so much that I lashed out and I hated that even more. Finally, I just curled up and didn't get out of bed or change out of my pajamas. I had chosen to wallow in feeling sorry for myself. I lay in my puddle of misery with no one really knowing what to do with me. My family had never seen me like this and really didn't know what to do. Eileen came to visit while I was in this state. She was brought upstairs to my bedroom. I was thinking: "Why did she come? Who is she? What does she want? What does she know about what I am going through?" The first thing Eileen said to me was that my bed was low and she didn't like to look down on people when she spoke to them. I thought that was odd, coming from her, who often stood at a podium or pulpit. I had two chairs in a corner in my room and she beckoned for me to join her there. Obediently, I got up and joined her. Eileen offered me the books she had brought me and started to read out loud from one of them. This is what she read:

Ida, The One Who Suffers
Whatever happens to me,
Has already happened to Ida, the one who suffers,
Only worse,
And with complications,
And the surgeon says it's a miracle she survived,
And her team of lawyers is suing for half a million,
And her druggist gave a gasp when he read the prescription,
And her husband never saw such courage,
Because (though it may seem like bragging) she's not a complainer,
Which is why the nurse was delighted to carry her bedpan,
And her daughter flew in from the sit-in to visit,
And absolute strangers were begging to give blood donations,
And the man from the Prudential even had tears in his eyes,
Because (though it may sound like bragging) everyone loves her,
Which is why both of her sisters were phoning on day rates from Denton,
And her specialist practically forced her to let him make house calls,
And the lady who cleans insisted on coming in Sundays,
And the cousins have cancelled the Cousins Club meeting,

And she's almost embarrassed to mention how many presents
Keep arriving from girlfriends who love her all over the
country,
All of them eating their hearts out with worry for Ida,
The one who suffers
The way other people
Enjoy.

(Author Unknown)

Not long into Ida, I started to laugh. I had experienced people around me complain so grandly when they had an earache or a headache or a toe ache, nothing as serious as cancer. I was judging and thinking that people around me were putting on the victim act like Ida. Soon, that judgment backfired and I was looking right back at me as the one being like Ida. By this time, I was already laughing and was able to start laughing at myself. That was the finest lesson about laughter that I could have been given. I share Ida with fondness whenever the moment is right. Learn to laugh at yourself, it is good medicine.

Dr. Siegel talks about joy and flat out laughter. In his book, *Love, Medicine and Miracles*, he talks about humor being the best medicine against cancer. He tells a story about a woman who's rather large. I forget her name, so I'll call her Doris. Doris had lung cancer and attended the Exceptional Cancer Patient group run by Dr. Siegel on a regular basis. From his description, I imagined Doris arriving at the group every week wearing the most inappropriate outfits like shorts, open midriff tops in clashing colors and always wearing a hat. Her hats were ones she made herself out of scraps and recycled junk and they were outrageous. One day, she announced to the group that her latest lung X-rays showed no sign of cancer whatsoever. After a time of joyous celebration, Dr. Siegel announced the reason why her cancer had shrunk was that no self-respecting cancer could live under the outrageous hats and outfits that she wore. Doris had scoffed and laughed at the cancer, in its face, by wearing her crazy outfits. She didn't take the cancer seriously enough to give it any foothold in her body. Laughter can be a powerful thing. Having a sense of humor about your cancer can help you heal.

After reading that story, while I was having chemo, I decided that if I lost my hair, I was going to walk around bald with a butterfly tattooed on the back of my head. That was many years ago when only old sailors and convicts had tattoos. I didn't lose all my hair, so I couldn't get the tattoo, but the humor of visualizing myself with a tattoo on the back of my head helped me get through chemo with a sense of amusement of how I would stick my middle finger in the air at cancer. The story of Doris and her outfits possibly having had an effect on her cancer has induced me to consciously dress to kill because I dress to kill cancer.

If you allow it to, cancer has the power to do many things with your emotions. It can evoke every negatively charged emotion and it can rob you of the joys of living. Your mind has the power to regain control if you identify what you are really feeling, naming the emotion and spending time with the emotion to understand how it works in your life. Your mind is powerful in thinking past the emotion and making unexpected connections for you. It will help you process what you can do for yourself and lead to better self-control over your emotions and the cancer.

You saw that laughter and joy are an essential part of life and beating cancer and you learned that even when you least feel like laughing, a habit of putting yourself into a situation that exposes you to laughter and joy will help these emotions return to their rightful place in your life again.

Learning about emotions helps create your perspectives about life. What you have already experienced in life adds to the way that you see life in general. Your attitude or mindset is a key part of how you overcome cancer. Mindset and its importance in dealing with cancer is what I'll discuss next.

Chapter 4

MINDSET

~

We've talked about the emotions, now let's talk about attitude. In this chapter I'll show you five things that influence attitude and discuss some practices that can help shift your mindset to a better place.

Viktor Frankl, M.D., Ph.D., in his book, *Man's Search for Meaning,* talks about people who give up on life are people without a sense of purpose. Purpose gives you a reason to live and it shapes your attitude towards life. No one can take away your attitude from you. When faced with cancer your positive attitude is challenged to its limit, You have to change your attitude to break out of the caged feeling that you may be experiencing. One way is through asking for help. If you find yourself saying to people who are trying to help you that they don't understand because they don't know what it's like to have cancer, you are choosing to stay trapped behind the attitude of being a victim. You're thinking very small. You can expand your thinking and change your attitude.

Here are five things that you can do about your attitude:

One: Seek joy. Joy seems to have been taken away from you. You've been robbed of joy when diagnosed with cancer. It's a bit like the glad emotion thing - that you have to go out and fake it until you make it. You have seek joy in small things every day. Search for things that make you happy or read things that will show you joy again. For example, you could read a daily motivational snippet. In the beginning you may hate this exercise and not want to do it. Force yourself to do this daily and develop the habit of seeking joy. Developing a joyous attitude about life will help you live through this. Find a daily motivational quote to inspire you and make you look outside of yourself. I read a story a day out of *Chicken Soup for the Soul*. It helped me look beyond myself and I started seeing the marvelous generosity and love that is in the world. There are many, many motivational books with short stories and quotes to help lift you up.

Two: Include others. When I say include others, you have to seek out people who are going to be truly supportive of you. I had a good friend who was diagnosed with a chronic disease other than cancer. I had no clue what it was but what she described sounded awful. I must have had a look on my face that said, "Oh my God. What's going to happen to you? I feel so sorry for you." She looked me straight in the eye and she said, "Stop that! You have that look on your face like you feel sorry for me. This disease is not going to change who I am." She said, "I don't want your sympathy. The only place I want to find sympathy is in the dictionary, between shit and syphilis." That truth still cracks me up and I repeat it often.

I don't want sympathy either. When I was going through my experiences with cancer the people who approached me with sympathy annoyed me the most. They seemed to feel sorry for themselves about knowing someone with cancer and they showed pity. I didn't want pity as I do not see sympathy as being productive. When you include others to help you fight cancer, scruitinize them, observe them and include those that really love you – warts and all. These are the people who love what's inside you, not what's happening inside you.

Three: You have to be able to reach outward. Reaching outward means that although you have to build those inner resources, you also have to reach out to others, so that they can share your experience in a positive light and you've got to give to others. Dr. Siegel talks about the altruistic mind, or altruistic mindset, of the cancer patient. The more you do for others, the more you heal yourself.

Four: Be grateful every day. What are you grateful for, right now? You're still alive, so there's one small thing. I'm sure that you can find the other things that you are grateful for. It might be the sunshine or a sunrise like the one I woke up to this morning. The sunrise was behind me, but looking out of my window, all I could see were bands of pale pink and blue. It was spectacular and I spent a moment feeling grateful for seeing the beauty in front of me. Your gratitude may be for the aroma of coffee or the smell of a fresh flower. There are so many things that, if you put our mind to it, you can find to be grateful for. Small things in ordinary places can make you smile, feel alive and experience gratitude. I do not drink coffee, however I love the aroma of coffee being ground. Sometimes I would catch a whiff of freshly ground coffee in the supermarket near the coffee aisle. It would make me pause and breathe deeply, happy for the experience. You do not have to find major things to be grateful for. Simple things will come to you more frequently, so you will have many opportunities to enjoy these small things and feel gratitude often.

Five: Be intentional. Every day, wake up and tell yourself that you are going to live today and how you're going to live. The more you make it a conscious endeavor to live life, the more life's richness will be restored and cancer will no longer have power over you.

When you want to generate energy and joy, remember this quote from Brendon Burchard, author of *The Motivational Manifesto*: "The power plant does not have energy, it generates an energy." The same thing applies to joy, that enthusiasm for life, that the intentionality of living life and the gratitude for life. Generate it.

Changing your mindset is about daily practices. In later chapters I will give you several practices to help you find the ones you prefer. You have to choose the ones that are going to rescue you from the fear, the anguish and anxiety initially. Those practices will change later to make you more robust and forthright and live life more generously, with yourself and other people. The practices are not cast in stone, but there are some that will become your foundation. Your foundational practices have to be done daily. For example, journal daily, visualize healing from cancer several times a day, meditate and be still once or twice daily. Add a guided imagery practice to your meditation time. These are healing practices. Become conscious of them at all times, so for example, every time you go out and you exercise, you walk and you're walking that cancer right out of your life. You give yourself mantras as you do things that are repetitive, to change your mindset, to give you that power and the strength again.

Visualization is a very powerful tool that can help you to change your mindset. Visualization can be done during everyday activities, like when you're in the shower for example. As you feel the water run off your body, you can visualize it washing away the cancer. When you're running water to wash your hands, visualize the water is washing off the cancer. When you're running water to wash dishes, your hair or watering the garden, you can visualize taking a moment to be conscious of the cancer being washed out of you.

I'll talk more about practices like guided imagery and visualizations, and other things that you can do on a daily basis later in the book. I want to introduce these thoughts to you now so that you can start having control over cancer and what your mind does with the cancer.

Often, when I'm feeling miserable or when I'm feeling defeated, I know it is what I call "my cancer brain" that is talking to me. I have to consciously do something to defeat that cancer brain every day. You can too. All you have to do is to start simple mind practices and habits to change your mindset.

Here is an idea to get you started. Think of your current state of mind. Sit with it without judging it. Write it down or draw a picture of it. Think of the mindset that you would prefer to have. What does that look like, what does it feel like and how would you be if you had that preferred mindset? Write your thoughts down about your ideal mindset or draw the ideal state of mind.

Look at what you have drawn or written and think of one thing you can do to shift closer to your desired mindset. Write that thing down in the present tense, as though it is already happening. Practice hearing yourself acting on this new belief. For example:

If your current state of mind is fear and you cannot see beyond cancer and that every ache and pain is evidence of more cancer, think about what you would rather be thinking. Could it be that you would rather be thinking that your body is normal, the aches and pains are normal and have nothing to do with cancer taking over your body? Practice saying out loud: My body has normal responses to life and I am living life normally with all the energy that I desire. Practice saying your positive state of mind statement daily; say it out loud so your subconscious hears it. If you are willing to take a risk, say it out aloud while looking at yourself in the mirror at least twice a day.

In this chapter you were presented with ways to look at your attitude towards life with cancer and your mindset. It is tough to make an attitude shift when cancer is a reality, however the shift from being a victim to being victorious is life changing. The way to change your mindset is not complicated; it takes a little practice every day. Hearing yourself affirm that your life is what you want it to be will shift your mindset into a belief system that you can put all your energy behind.

Next we'll talk about making conscious choices on how you want to be living your life, building on the concepts you have already learned and adding practices that establish a full and meaningful life.

Chapter 5

PLAN
TO LIVE CONSCIOUSLY

―――――――― ～ ――――――――

This chapter will discuss how to take the conscious decision to live beyond a mere decision and will teach you simple practices to achieve conscious living with a positive mindset. The goal is to beat cancer. Whenever you set goals, you have to have clarity to achieve the goal. Achieving clarity with a goal like beating cancer can be a challenge because your mind is immediately flooded with thoughts, ideas and doubts, and can easily lead to overwhelm. If you are reading this book to help a loved one, you might be able to help shift the numbness of overwhelm by helping your loved one to take small steps towards the ultimate goal. Notice, I did not say kill or eradicate cancer. Often all you have to do is to learn to live with it until you figure out what your cure will be. So for now, while still having to live with the cancer present, it is important to live consciously.

Here are some habits to help you live more consciously.

Life-giving habits

Visualization and guided imagery

The quickest habit to establish to help restore hope is visualization. I spoke a bit about it in the previous chapter when talking about the mind. I see guided imagery and visualization as a life-restoring habit. Actively imagining what you want your body needs to do to deal with the cancer can help restore control over the thoughts and fears and help to regain control over cancer. Visualization can do both. Think about what you "see" you have to do to rid yourself of cancer. What does your body need, what does it need help with in order to kill the cancer cells? Now think of that thing that your body should be doing better and turn it into something you can visualize.

O. Carl Simonton, M.D., Stephanie Matthews-Simonton and James Creighton wrote the book, *Getting Well Again,* specifically for cancer patients. It is a highly recommended book about guided imagery and the mind-body connection to healing. The Simontons wrote about this many years ago and were even able to teach children how to visualize their cancer being eaten away by the body's fighter cells. They cite the example of a child with a brain tumor who was taught to imagine a cat sitting in front of a bowl of dry cat food pellets. The child had to visualize the cat eating the pellets until the bowl was completely clean once or twice a day. The child's tumor disappeared.

Martin Rossman, M.D., in his book *Guided Imagery for Self-Healing,* talks about guided imagery rather than visualization. I tend to use the terms interchangeably because I am a visual thinker. The difference between the two is that in guided imagery you are eliciting responses to questions without necessarily having to "see" these in your imagination as with visualization. Some people cannot visualize. Guided imagery can be even more powerful in fighting cancer than merely visualizing. Exploring your responses to questions about your cancer in a guided imagery is a real way to come up with your way to beat cancer. Drs. Rossman and Siegel suggest having a conversation in your head with a "trusted advisor." Put the question to your advisor about what you should do about a certain aspect of your treatment or a new approach you heard about. That inner conversation can be extremely powerful and enlightening, helping you find answers you didn't think you had, but also giving you a powerful way to imagine yourself fighting cancer successfully during your meditations.

I mostly used visualization and had two favorite cancer-fighting visualizations to tell my immune system what I wanted it to do. One was using the Pac-Man game. Pac-Man was the symbol for my entire immune system gobbling up cancer cells as it went. I could even hear the noise that the game made every time Pac-Man scored a victory and the target disappeared. When all the targets were cleared out and only green lines of the maze remained, my Pac-Man turned around and gobbled up all the green lines until my imaginary TV screen was completely black and cleansed of any vestiges of cancer. That was always so satisfying! Try it.

My second visualization was of amoeba-like, chemo-carrying cells with little garbage bags over their shoulders marching through my veins, absorbing cancer cells into their garbage bags as they went. When the bags were full, my little army of cells marched to the huge, exceedingly hot furnace in the bowels of my being and threw each bag into the flames to be destroyed completely. Then off they went to start the process over again. I even had a tune that went along with their work - it was the Seven Dwarf's song from the Disney movie, *Snow White,* "Hey ho, Hey ho, it's off to work I go." And you're welcome for my getting that song stuck in your head now. Visualizations like these can take three to five minutes and can be hugely empowering. Try to do them three or more times a day.

Dr. Siegel is a strong proponent of guided imagery and visualization, using a slightly different technique when focusing on the cancer is too difficult. Here is my version of his guided imagery: Visualize a place where you can be completely happy and at peace. I visualized a gazebo in the middle of a beautiful garden. Add as much color and detail into your special place and try to include all your senses.

What does it look like, what do you see around you, what are the shapes and shadows? What does it smell like? Where would you be sitting or reclining in this place? What would make it comfortable and pleasing to you and make it your very own creation? How does it make you feel physically and emotionally to be there? What are the sounds of your special place? You could add gentle music to go with this visualization.

Now, if there were significant people who you want to share this place with, visualize them being with you, hugging you, supporting and loving you. This is a place of joy and of healing for your body. Stay there as long as you like and soak up the good, uplifting feelings that this place allows you to experience. If you like, you can allow a healing golden light to enter from above that surrounds you with health, joy and life. When you are ready, build a bridge to take you back to your everyday place and savor the moment of bringing back the feeling of peace with you. I suggest that you mark this page or record your voice guiding you through the imagery and use it whenever you need some help in getting to focus on the practice.

Remember the endorphins that the brain releases? As a result of the visualization, these endorphins are released and are now telling your immune system to speed up. Block time to do your guided imagery or visualization at least twice a day. The cleansing water visualization or other cancer-healing imagery can be done almost everywhere and anytime. While driving, I used to imagine the moving traffic as smoothly operating immune cells moving to their destinations to successfully kill off cancer cells. Developing a consciousness that you can fight cancer while doing anything is pretty empowering.

With all the exercises and practical suggestions so far, you might be feeling that you won't have time to do much more. Well, maybe, but remember that the cancer is at it 24/7 and your immune system needs all the help you can give it as often and for as long as you can every day. Be realistic with your available time and fit something new into your day every day. Being consciously active against the cancer is a fine way to keep your cancer brain from robbing you of good thoughts. Keep your brain busy and your emotions will be easier to manage too.

Writing and drawing

A great habit to have is keeping a gratitude journal. I know that sounds crazy when you might still be struggling with anger, fear and sadness; however, when I have done this, even grudgingly, I have felt an emotional shift. It is like a reality check helping you to get to the root of life and what makes you happy. My journal was all pretty much about the sadness and fears initially, but every now and then I was able to find something to write about that I was truly thankful for. Those are moments that I cherished most and am glad that I captured them.

Initially it took me some time to get to the gratitude part of journaling, but I did start writing daily thoughts, emotions, fears and successes. Successes led to writing about my gratitude. From reading and learning about how to be a successful leader, I have learned that many successful people keep a gratitude journal. They say that it keeps them sane, humble and balanced.

When fighting cancer we need all the help we can get to remain sane. I'm not so sure about humble, because my arrogance and stubbornness worked to my advantage when I needed those and to my disadvantage at times as well. Maybe I should have written more so that I could have learned more humility and balance. We certainly need balance because the internal imbalance is what threw our healthy physiology off to begin with.

So start writing. It doesn't matter if you don't know what to write; write about that. When you have those six words on the page, express your gratitude that you won't have me standing over you expecting that you write something. Remember the part about naming the emotion? This is a good place to start writing. Make a list of all your emotions, add some reasons why you feel them and voila! - You have started writing a journal about your experience with cancer. Write down your thoughts about your sanity and cancer. Is there any gratitude you feel there? Write about humility and how you experience that and what you are grateful for in humility. Write about what balance means to you and what you think needs to change in order for you to experience more balance. Writing about everyday things and your gratitude for them is a very healing, wholesome exercise.

Drawing is another expressive way to deal with cancer to shift your mindset. Dr. Siegel asks his patients to draw themselves, their cancer and their cure. I remember drawing myself cowering and looking up at a huge spider hanging over my head and an even bigger injection needle right in front of me. I am really scared of needles and injections, less so spiders, so what I had drawn was myself being terrorized by the treatment more than disease! Seeing that reality drove me to want to change the picture and my mindset. So I redrew the picture to put the cancer in its place as a tiny spider, my cure and me working together to give me the muscle to stomp out the cancer. Had I not drawn the original picture, I would not have seen how afraid I had been of chemo. It helped me to do something to change that perspective a little.

Later on, with another cancer diagnosis, I drew myself, not alone, this time, but with a group of supporters to help me. The clump of cowering cancer cells in my drawing had no chance, they looked trapped and afraid anticipating their demise as an army of boots marched over them. This drawing was a powerful message to my subconscious. It helped me feel that I could stomp out cancer with all the love and support that I had.

Other things that you can draw are the obstacles that you have for seeing your cure. What do these obstacles represent? What do they look like? How big are they in relation to you? Now draw your Super-Self leaping over the obstacles in some way. My biggest obstacle was a brick wall. For me, it was symbolic of no one listening to my needs or communicating with me other than telling me what I would or would not be doing to deal with the cancer. The drawing I did to depict overcoming my obstacle was of me dismantling the wall brick by brick. As I drew the fallen bricks around me, I started seeing who I had to talk to, who would support me and who I needed to seek out for additional support. I became more open about talking about my cancer in some circles I had kept separate because they were "professional" circles. My belief was that I should keep a strict separation between personal issues and professional discussions, so, for a long time, I didn't disclose my diagnosis to a group of fellow coaches. After drawing the barriers, I saw that I was putting many of these up myself. I started opening up, shared the situation I was in with my coaching peers, and through that, I was introduced to one of the most significant people whose wisdom saved my life. I referred to her as my "cancer coach" initially, but soon she became my "wholeness coach." Her name is Jeanette Bronee', a nutritionist, author and speaker who has done TED talks about health. Look her up at www.pathforlife.com. Had I not done the drawing of my barriers to my cure, I would have remained silent about the cancer. Had I not followed Jeanette's advice about toxic relationships, I would not be here to write this book.

An interesting thing happens when writing or drawing about cancer, your fears, your cure, your aspirations and your future after cancer, it helps you gain new insights and helps you to process these. This is an amazing way to put things in perspective. It helps you examine your attitude or misgivings, see what it is that you need to face and deal with, or reveals strategies and determination to live well with cancer or to get rid of it.

A healthy respect for your mind and good strategies for understanding how it works inside your head comes from expressing your affirmations daily. It energizes the fight or it forces you to look for support when you know you cannot do it alone every day. Write or draw daily and fight the despair and overwhelm by processing this cancer every day. If you teach your mind to do this, your body will follow and learn to do so as well. Once you have done your initial drawings, revealing what you want for your life, draw and write about ways you will celebrate life.

While I was living in Indiana and had started becoming more vocal about cancer and sharing my journey, I was invited to speak at a women's gathering. The theme for my talk was "Living Life Loudly." The audience was a group of primarily very quiet, conservative and obedient women. The talk flopped totally. To add to the discomfort, I added the shit and syphilis story. That was not received well either. What I learned from this experience is that living life loudly might work for me, but everyone has to find his or her own motivation for living. Writing and drawing about how you want to celebrate life, as it is every day, could help you find the inner drive to get you through today. You do not have to be ambitious about seeing beyond today – I do urge you to live today!

In this chapter you learned that you can make conscious choices about how you guide your thinking, how you can introduce movement into your life and how drawing and writing can broaden your perspectives and add healing practices to daily life. These practices bring us out of unconscious numbness and into consciousness again. They offer us ways to shift our automatic responses to chosen thoughts and visualizations about how we want life to be, enriching our minds again with pleasant experiences and giving respite from the difficulties of living with cancer.

What you just learned were strategies that helped me and other survivors cope and go beyond just coping, into a life more richly lived because of bringing conscious choice back into life again.

In the next chapter I'll focus on your team of healers and consciously making decisions about who, what type of healers you want to include on your team and the expectations you can have of effective team members who support you in living your life your way.

Chapter 6

CHOOSE YOUR TEAM OF HEALERS CONSCIOUSLY

———————⌁———————

Chapter 6 is about not settling for the first doctors who identified the cancer as being the obvious choice for deciding your medical treatment. We will explore the possibilities of second and third opinions, as well as informed advice from alternative and holistic practitioners from any discipline, which may have an attraction for you. This chapter is about exploring your options.

The problem with being diagnosed with cancer is that you are put into a situation where someone else takes over the decisions being made over your life. What will put you back in control right away is deciding consciously that *you* are the head of your healing team. You have to have people on your team with whom you can be open, ask questions without being intimidated and to help you remember the questions you wanted to ask in the first place. Your team can consist of family, your best friend, a trusted primary care physician or general practitioner (GP), a naturopath, nutritionist, exercise coach counselor or support group in addition to the oncologists who have entered your life.

Actively searching for this team took me three months. Four doctors either resigned or were fired until I found the best oncologist I could have ever asked for. He immediately gave me hope that I should continue my search for other healers as he helped me look at the medical options other than chemotherapy and start the treatment. He was referred to me by my GP who had seen me get angry and feeling that I was being treated like a brainless idiot by the current oncologist, whose behavior told me that her research was really all she cared about and finding out that she had made me undergo an unnecessary surgery. Here is the story: When I announced my concern about an itchy boob to the treating oncologist, she immediately sent me for a skin biopsy, which surgically removed a section of my breast tissue to find out what my GP could have identified by looking, listening and asking me questions. The weekend before my oncology appointment, I had been weeding in my garden. Because my GP was familiar with the area I lived in, he was immediately suspicious that I had a case of poison ivy. However, I only told him about the situation after I had already had the biopsy and was waiting for him to receive the results. It took more than a week and many attempts for him to finally receive the full biopsy report from the oncologist. The result, in the words on the report: Evidence of contact dermatitis, as in poison ivy.

I tell you this story to highlight that you probably have the right support in your back yard. When we deal with cancer, we do not always need the oncologist to take over all our medical decisions. This experience taught me that the specialist didn't know me, could not put things into perspective by knowing my lifestyle and my GP could. He knew that I loved gardening, knew the area I lived in and the high likelihood of my itchy, cancerous boob having nothing to do with the cancer at all. Instead, my health insurance and I were made to pay for an unnecessary surgical procedure and lab tests, which could all have been avoided if I went to my GP first. I had always seen him as my trusted medical advisor, but had been sidetracked by the importance I had given the esteemed cancer center's oncology team. This experience solidified his role as my trusted advisor again and I benefitted from his advice many times during that journey through cancer. When I moved to Portland, Oregon, my first quest was to find a new doctor who I could turn to for sound advice and support. I used a service called nurse navigators. They listened to who I needed, what kind of person I was and suggested some names of medical and naturopathic doctors in the area who they thought might be a good fit for me. I have been blessed with superb doctors who care for and who hear me. Since then I have met other people going through cancer who have been very happy with their doctors who have a very different approach to mine. The common thread, however, is that they listened to their hearts when selecting their healers.

One of my current healers, who I believe has saved my life from a cardiac struggle, came from a referral through a business networking event. Had I not explored that suggestion, my quality of life would not be what it is today!

Here are things to think about when assembling your healing team:

Who do you want on your healing team? You presumed that the doctor who read your test results and diagnosed the cancer should be on your team, but is that person the right person to support and guide you and be your mentor through your entire journey? If not, then you have to explore whom the right person is to be your right-hand person. Never forget that you are the head of the team. The doctors, naturopaths, homeopaths and Chinese medicine specialists who you invite to be part of your cure are there to guide you and help you make decisions that are important to you by adding their knowledge and perspectives. They can give you options and resources. Don't let them prescribe your treatment without finding out everything you should know before you say yes to the course of treatment or strategy. It has to feel right to you and your immediate, trusted team members.

I do believe that the right team will show up for you. All you have to do is be prepared to explore options and to listen. There is a fable about a man who was diagnosed with cancer who fervently prayed to God for a cure. His doctor sent him to an oncologist who said to the man, "With chemotherapy, I can cure your cancer." The man refused chemo and said that he was praying to God for a cure. So the oncologist referred the man to a radiation oncologist who said to the man, "I can cure your cancer with radiation," to which the man replied, "I am praying to God, He will cure me." The radiation specialist referred the man to a naturopath who said, "Take these supplements and your tumor will shrink." Again the man responded with the same reply. The naturopath referred the man to a dietician renowned for curing cancer with diet. Again he refused. Finally, the man died. When he saw God he asked God why he hadn't cured him. God said: "I sent you an oncologist, a radiation specialist, a naturopath and a dietician and you refused. What more could I have done?"

Because I believed that I would find my cure, I also believed that I would find the right team of healers. Every time they have shown up when I have needed them. All you have to do is to put the request "out there" in the universe by writing it down, focusing on that daily and then be open to who shows up.

Choose the rest of your Holistic team consciously.

Don't ask your doctors about alternative therapies; this is not their field of expertise. Many oncologists see the benefits of a holistic approach to cancer, but usually cannot refer you to practitioners outside of medicine because they typically do not know who is out there. Ask your friends and family. Ask your extended support group. Most of these referrals come by word-of-mouth. The Internet is a great tool; however, you have to vet what is being talked about. A first step to assembling the rest of your healing team might be to assign research to one or two of your people. Most people around us are feeling lost and useless. Give them something meaningful to do and they step right up. The Cancer Centers of America are a great resource for finding alternative practitioners. I found my nutritionist there and we had phone consultations. I had not met her in person until she came to do a talk locally about fighting cancer with your fork. Her name is Kim Dalzell; she has written several books about the nutritional approach to fighting cancer. The one I read is *Challenge Cancer and Win.* It had a chapter on each different type of cancer and her recommended diets for each.

My friend who has become my role model has found numerous recipe books and cancer-fighting diet books, too many to mention here. Do your research or get one of your team members to search for books. The ones that attract you will most likely have the strategies you are willing to follow. The authors of these books become your team members by extension. Discuss the approaches with your holistic team so that they are aware of your inclination and approach. If they are not familiar with the particular supplement or regime that they might suggest, find out if there is anything that will interfere with the strategies that you have already chosen. Cancer recovery does not come from a single approach; several things can contribute to your healing when applied at the same time. Listen and follow your instincts.

Don't exclude anything until you get a feel for what the approach has done for cancer and to what degree has it been successful. I have heard of people with cancer finding Reiki, acupuncture and many different diet and supplement programs to be useful for reducing their fear, helping them relax and helping them get well again. You will learn about these as you go along, but don't think you have to have your full team assembled right now. As I said before, you do have time. Focus your attention on what you think needs to be done first, and then add as you go along. Get family members to do the research for you but don't let them push you to do anything that doesn't feel right to you. Be open-minded, though; you never know what might be very useful in your healing approach. You might hear of something that sounds totally bizarre, but it may be appealing to you. I was told about an aloe vera supplement that others had debunked without my knowledge. I put my faith in this supplement as my cure and it worked! It may not work for me now, because now I have doubts about it's clinical effectiveness after reading articles questioning the supplement company's claims. You have to believe in your approach wholeheartedly in order for the right message to be received subconsciously to trigger your body's healing ability. If I had doubts about the vegan diet, it would not have worked. If I had doubts about adding hormone-free, organic animal products, to my diet, those would have worked against me. If I didn't trust my naturopathic doctor, her supplement regime would not work. Your belief in the approaches you choose is usually based on the relationship of trust that you have for the person giving you advice.

Totally unrelated things about coping with the side effects of having cancer treatment might be attractive to you. Explore what might be important to you especially if it could result in a dramatic change to your body image. No matter how the oncologist tried to pressure me into having a radical mastectomy, I stalled, waiting to hear other alternatives. You can wait a week or more before jumping into a treatment approach that makes significant changes to your body and your self-image. Think about what you value about your body, your image and your emotional response to changes that you face.

My sister-in-law said that she wished she had known about having eyebrows tattooed under her own eyebrows before she had started with chemo. Having eyebrows was important to her. You are not advised to go for tattooing during chemo because you become more vulnerable to infection. I have decided to share this with people because it might make a difference to their mood during chemo, especially when they look in the mirror after losing their hair. One of my friends had a perm before starting chemo. Her thinking was that if her hair was going to fall out, it may as well be curly and she would enjoy her new look while it lasted. Her hair didn't fall out. The reverse is true too. A woman who had the same surgeon and oncologist as I, having the same medical approaches, had beautiful hair, which she was terrified she would lose. She was a pathologist and had researched the type of chemo we were being given and all its effects on the cells of the body so she was convinced that we would lose our hair. She did, I didn't. I decided to experiment with scarves and the idea of the butterfly tattoo before the hair loss started, and didn't lose enough hair to warrant the tattoo. Do not think that all useful information has to come from experts. My daughter Megan was playing with scarves with me one day soon after I started chemo and she was the person who ultimately came up with the best scarf design for me that made me feel pretty and confident while hiding the hair loss. I think Megan was three at the time. You never know whom your inspirations will come from to help you feel whole again while on this journey.

People who have been through the experience successfully can be a great support. They can help you through some of the tough times and they can tell you what to avoid. When all is said and done, though, you will be the one to discern who to follow and listen to and whose advice does not resonate with you. Beware those who are there to tell you more about the side effects than their good outcomes. Unfortunately, not every person who has gone through cancer comes out washed clean of his or her negativity.

This chapter was about deciding whom you trust and who will trust you and your decisions about the approaches you want to take for healing from cancer. It made you look at who you already have and who you might need to look for to complete your team. There is no definitive number or makeup of a perfect cancer-fighting team. No matter how your team takes shape, you are always the head of the team, making sure that the team works with you and supports your desires and aspirations about your cure or the way you want to live with cancer.

I hope that this has given you the confidence that your decisions are based on gathering the right people with the answers that seem right for you. There is no perfect life, but you can get so much more from life by not doubting your own instincts about what you are told regarding treatment, nutrition and other supportive therapies that make sense to you. Good team members can balance each other and help make your decisions feel right.

Next we will tackle what is a toxic environment for your thinking and what is a nurturing environment for your mind.

Chapter 7

CONSCIOUSLY CHOOSE YOUR ENVIRONMENT

Experiencing constant fear of what the environment is doing to you is not healthy. Cancer feeds off fear and cancer feeds fear. You're stuck between these two realities of this disease. However, there are choices you need to make about your environment for better air, better quality of water and better food from a better environment. These are all choices that you can make about your environment to help you improve your body's chance against cancer. You might not be able to improve all of the factors, but work on the ones you can improve.

The environment in most cities is toxic and you typically don't do anything to protect yourself until you have a medical condition to make you pay attention. Now is a good time to start paying attention. I'm not suggesting that you wear a full HAZMAT suit; you don't need to draw that much attention to yourself. Become aware of your rights as a citizen and what choices you have in the situation. I have a friend who became aware that the weed killer being sprayed along the roads in her area was highly toxic. She became a strong lobbyist to have the practice changed. When that didn't work, she moved to a healthier environment.

There is an additional environment people do not always think of, and that is the social environment. Look at this as well and become aware of the impact of your social environment has on your health. Relationships are a key factor to your success in this adventure. Significant people will be a huge help but you need to learn to recognize toxic people and relationships and how to set boundaries to support your wellbeing.

Start thinking about what you feel the chief toxins are in your life. Mine were sugar and relationships. Yes, people can be part of the toxic environment, so I say scrutinize everything around you and assess what seems to be toxic and what does not. Pay a lot of attention to the people who start paying attention to you since your diagnosis of cancer. They can be toxic as well. Not all "do-gooders" have pure intentions. Some of them have subconscious needs that they are not even aware of, but you need to be aware of the environment they create near you. Let me tell you a story about how my best friend and soul mate and I met.

In South Africa we typically would have to drive or walk our children to school. This meant that at the end of the school day there would be gatherings of parents waiting for their children. When I was diagnosed with cancer, somehow the gossipers knew all about it. People who I had never encountered before started coming up to me to ask how I was doing. When I answered that I was fine, the next question would be, "Tell me how you are *really* doing." Since I *really* didn't know them, I didn't see their interest as being genuine.

There was one woman in particular who was toxic. Her approach was to tell me all about another pupil's mother, Liz, who had leukemia and who, according to the gossip, was not doing well at all. Gossip Lady was way worse than Ida, gasping and stopping short of nothing to tell me, in detail, how bad Liz's blood tests were and that because Liz's husband had come to fetch the children from school, Liz had taken a turn for the worse. Gossip Lady took turns frequenting the gathering-place at the tree, where I usually waited for my daughters, and the gate where Liz picked her children up. When Gossip Lady positioned herself at the gate, Liz had the pleasure of hearing all about how poorly I was doing and that the chemo was taking its toll because my hair had become thin and wispy like the lady who volunteered at the school tuck shop. When Gossip Lady was at the tree, I heard all about Liz's decline in great detail. After a couple of weeks of this I finally asked who Liz was, got her full name and called her up. Liz's response when she heard who was calling was "Oh, I know all about every chemo you have had and how many hairs are left on your head!" I retorted that I knew her white blood cell count and the pallor of her skin. We laughed, met in person and became best friends. Our nicknames for each other became Skat or Skattie, meaning "treasure" in Afrikaans. My Skattie became my soul mate and will live in my heart forever as a healing presence. We weathered the storms of cancer and chemo together and shared the joys of our children and what life gave us, and we have a gossip to thank for that.

Our experience with Gossip Lady taught us that there were people we had to protect ourselves from. We nicknamed our gossip PD, short for Profit of Doom. It is important to recognize the PDs and to protect yourself from their toxicity. If Liz and I had not been able to support each other and develop our strategies for not allowing the gossip get to us, I think we would have been far more vulnerable to the toxicity of that experience.

Our PD had created such a web of lies about what was happening to me that, when I bumped into another school parent while shopping, the woman's jaw dropped and she turned white, as though she had seen a ghost. Once she composed herself, she told me that PD, who claimed that she was an intimate friend of mine, was telling people that I was close to death and how everyone should be praying for my daughters and husband. Instead of encountering me reposed in a coffin, the woman saw me jauntily going shopping in a bright turquoise dress and flowing scarf; nowhere close to the description being given by PD to anyone who would listen. The thing about PDs is that they feed off other people's distress and use it to get attention for their own sick needs. You might have cancer, but are not that sick. Protect yourself by avoiding them like the plague.

Situations can also be unintentionally toxic. I have a friend who recently decided to join a Bible study class. The focus was on disobedience and God's punishment for disobedience. At first she tried to be more obedient but soon realized that she had not been disobedient to begin with. Had she recognized that fact early in the discussions, she would have saved herself guilt and mental energy in her attempt to meet the standards of the study group. I see this as an example of an unintentional toxic environment. Choose your study and support groups carefully. Feeling guilty for not being good enough and that the cancer is your punishment is not healing. You are doing the best you can; there is no reason to add assumed burdens because of dogma or opinion. I was once asked to leave a support group run by a social worker at a Breast Center. I had told my story of beating cancer without chemo or radiation. My intention was to give women hope that they could survive, no matter what. The social worker felt that I was not supportive of the medical model, which she represented and that I was giving the women in the group "false hope." I was sorry to leave the group because I felt that I needed support too. Three women from the group, who were interested in alternatives to medical approaches contacted me and we became a support for each other, each of us following a slightly different version of a holistic approach. We are all still alive and well.

Create an interpersonal environment that serves you well by establishing good partners who have not been diagnosed with cancer as well. To be good partners, they will rely on you to educate them and to ask for what you need. You cannot assume that a family member or friend who has known you for many years knows what you need now. Just as your world was turned upside down, so has theirs. They need some guidance from you about your new needs.

The first things you can request from them is to help lift the burden of overwhelm. They can contribute to this by doing your research for you. If you can, be specific about what you are looking for. What kind of alternatives do you want to learn about? What dietary information do you want? A "cancer diet" might not be specific enough. If you haven't discovered the details of your thinking yet, let them do research in big areas, like supplements or diet and narrow down the options based on their findings. If you have done the journaling and drawing exercises, you might have an idea of what you specifically want to eliminate, add and do differently already. If you are starting from scratch, let them have free reign over that task and bring you small chunks of information with their impressions of whether they think it will be something you could put into practice or not. There is an overwhelming amount of information online about medical options, supportive therapies, wigs and reconstructive surgical options, to mention a few. Think about what you are really interested in knowing and let your partners help you sort through the irrelevant and unimportant for now.

Another thing you can ask of your team is to help protect you if you have a poisonous PD around you. Let your partners create a buffer for you by allowing you to escape from the PD's constant attention and inquiry.

There is an old African saying that, when in mourning, your energy should be devoted to mourning, not making major decisions. The family and community are expected to support mourners and protect them from any additional stress of everyday life. I think the same applies to dealing with cancer. You should not have to deal with irritations, aggravations and things that overwhelm you. Your energy is needed for healing and you could benefit from others giving you support when it comes to making everyday decisions.

Teach your support team how to support you emotionally. There are times that you just need to *be.* Being is a state of no activity, thought or conversation. It is a quiet place where you process life with cancer. Ask your partners to help support your need just to be. Healing happens when you allow yourself to be with the cancer in any way that it shows up for you. Your partners' silence and active listening are all you need in those moments. They will not know why you need silence unless you teach them how to be with you in your silence. They do not have to fill the air with cheery conversation. At times it is comforting just to sit in the sun alongside your friend and enjoy sharing that silent support.

Your friends and family may have strong opinions about what you should or should not do. The ultimate decision is yours. Help them understand this without judgment. If they learn to listen quietly and ask what is important to you at that moment, they will be true healers for you. You can't do this alone and neither can they. You are a team and teams get to learn an intimacy of insight and understanding that is very beautiful as well as restorative.

Treat your body as a partner in this process as well. That might sound odd, but think about it for a while. You are in the process of making conscious choices for your body. Body image is an integral part of your being. When cancer invades your body, you could feel immensely disappointed about your body's integrity and function; even its beauty. What do you think about your body now that you have cancer? What did you think of your body before cancer? How are these two thoughts different now? Write your thoughts in your journal. Feeling some negativity or disappointment is normal. You don't have to change everything to make a huge shift back to what was normal before. You do have to be kind to your body and not neglect it. This may become difficult if you choose a treatment that is hard on your body, but if you start with the right mindset, you will have less side effects and greater confidence in the outcomes. Partner with your body and listen to its needs throughout the process.

What needs to change about how you feel about your body right now? Start a visualization to imagine your body being healthy and whole. Add a part to your "happy place" visualization where you consciously see your body being perfect, with an efficient immune system and in superb health. Using positive affirmations out loud daily to endorse your state of mind and belief in your surviving cancer while doing what is best for your body gets the message to your brain frequently so that you can believe it throughout your body.

I know you may have thoughts that you are reading this too late to lengthen your lifespan. You can apply all of these techniques to help you live fully for as long as you are alive. Who knows, you might surprise your doctors and yourself. I know of two dramatic stories of people who outlived doctors' predictions. One was my best friend, Liz, who had been given six months to live and she lived for six years. The second was my friend and role model who was told she would probably not see the end of that summer after being diagnosed in April. She is still alive and about to celebrate her third year post-diagnosis. I believe with my entire being that no one can determine my expiration date and I defy any doctor who attempts to predict the end of my life. In fact, I feel so strongly about this that I have an immediate reaction when I hear people tell me that a doctor has told them that they only have a set time to live. Please ask doctors to refrain from these predictions. Life and how long you live is a personal thing. You either believe that this is between you and God or you believe that your lifespan is undetermined. Either way, live your life fully and the ending loses its meaning. I have survived three serious cancer diagnoses. Some doctors would have jumped to a conclusion about my mortality. Luckily, I protected myself from this by quickly telling the doctors that I did not want to hear their predictions. I know my thought processes well enough to know that I can be a dangerously obedient patient, to the point of dying at the expiration date falsely set by someone else. I believe that my story of survival is remarkable because I have chosen to live, not die as predicted.

This section focused on your mind and how to regain control of the emotions, the behaviors and environments that may have contributed to your body allowing cancer to grow inside you. I discussed ways to regain control of your mind and ways to make choices that will impact how you are treated, by whom and how you lead your team to support your healing pathway. By journaling, drawing and using visualizations you can shift your mindset from one of fear and loss of any control to having control over how you think of cancer and how your life will be from now on. You have a set of principles that will help guide you beyond the limiting thoughts cancer forces upon you to more enlightened ways of thinking about who you are now that you have cancer and what you will do about it.

Next we are going to tackle the realities of your body with cancer and what it needs from you in order to restore its ability to kill cancer cells and to have energy for life again.

SECTION 2

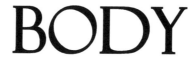

BODY

Chapter 8

YOUR BODY

We are about to embark on the part of the book that most non-cancer people like to focus on exclusively - your body. The focus on the corporal will make you feel that you have to slash and burn your body in order to punish your cells or shock them straight again. Not so. This chapter is going to show you how to be mindful of what your body needs and how you relate to your body to give it the tools to survive and do well.

No one needs to remind you that your body has weird cells that you would rather not have inside you. The good news is that this thing you call a body is really a magical healing machine. If you have cut yourself or broken a bone, you know what I'm talking about. The doctor may have stitched the cut or immobilize the bone, but it was your own cells that healed the skin, closed the cut and made it look normal again. The same applies to a broken bone. It was your body that healed the bone naturally inside you without any help from outside, except to stop you from moving the broken bits around by putting a cast around the limb to protect it from movement.

If the body can do that, why not heal cancer? I believe that it can. With the right mindset, even if it is still evolving, you can enhance the process that your body already knows but may have forgotten. Using the powerful tool of your mind you can teach your body to deal with cancer. I have done this twice without any significant medical interventions, so I know it is possible. I had chemo and radiation with my first bout of cancer, but I refused chemo, surgery or radiation the second time, and the third time I was diagnosed, my oncologist just put me back on a hormone blocker that I had voluntarily stopped three years earlier. My blood tests and scans show no evidence of cancer three years post diagnosis.

What did I do? I believed in my body's ability to fight disease, but I was also aware that I had neglected giving my body the right tools to be as efficient as it could be. I wanted to survive cancer, decided that my body was capable of it and did all I could to convince myself of the fact. And I sought a little help from the people around me who I trusted.

Your body has cancer. Now what? A way to start understanding what your body needs is to question your real understanding of your body, your relationship with it and how you see your body in your future. Some questions to ask yourself: How do you understand what that means in terms of your body and its function? What would the equal and opposite condition for your body be? Put differently, what do you want for your body?

How will you protect it and how do you think you can enhance its healing capacity?

Create a mind map of all the things you need in order for your body to get rid of the cancer cells. I started you off doing a mind map in an earlier chapter, but if you are still unclear, here is some instruction. A mind map is a creative process used for capturing all the random thoughts that occur to you on a topic so you can see all of them on one sheet of paper. It will help you start to organize thoughts into something more understandable and less random. Start with a blank sheet of paper – a big one if you have it. Write the word cancer in the center of the page and circle it. Around that core word add all the thoughts about what cancer means to your body, its potential cures, the medical and other resources you want to explore and habits you want to stop or start. All these words in bubbles of their own, radiating out from the center, will start to make sense. Categories will emerge. You will be able to connect categories and individual thoughts with lines that connect them to the main concept and to each other.

Plan to have a messy looking mind map; it is exactly what the cellular connections inside your brain look like. Lots of different ideas all connecting and reconnecting to help you make sense of what you think your body needs to do its job. Now you can start seeing themes and thoughts that make sense to you and those thoughts that make more important connections to healing cancer for you. It will help you decide what to do first, second, together or not at all. It will help you see a path towards counteracting the cancer, how to protect your body and how to enhance its normal functions. Use the mind map to make a list of key concepts and categories that are important for you to heal your body from cancer. Prioritize from this list what is most important to you right now and what may become the focus of your healing later. Creating a plan for your body's health will become clearer by using this method of sifting through all the information and thoughts.

Three healing options to explore

Medical.

Looking at cancer treatments from the perspective of being the patient is overwhelming. But remember that your team of doctors is there to help you make sense of what they are offering you. You have to know that it is OK for you to ask lots of questions and even ask the same ones over and over. You have already heard of chemo, radiation or surgery, but that does not mean that you understand the implications for your own body. What does all of that mean to you? Ask. Ask all the simplest questions and ask the more difficult ones. This is the only way to gather information that can make understanding what to do and what to prepare your body for.

Some doctors are not used to patients asking questions and can feel threatened, thinking that you are challenging their wisdom. Ask anyway. I had an oncologist who was 6 foot 4 inches tall and one day, when I had asked questions he didn't like, he stood up, leaned across the desk and spoke down to me like I was a disobedient child. That was tough as I was more than halfway through my chemo when this incident happened and didn't feel like I had the option of changing doctors at that stage of treatment. I never asked any questions after that and felt a total disconnect with this doctor and to my treatment. I started having more severe side effects. Luckily my GP was a wise saint and he supported me, asked questions on my behalf or sought the answers from other colleagues. What put this experience into perspective for me was someone who asked me if I knew the difference between God and a doctor. The answer is God doesn't have to pretend to be a doctor. After that my oncologist was referred to, tongue-in-cheek, as "my god the doctor." It helped me deal with the rest of my encounters with him.

This experience helped me decide that I would never be put into the situation of a poor relationship with a doctor again. It did not stop me from asking doctors questions. I just became more discerning about who I would have as my physician so that I would get the answers I needed.

Make a list of questions about your medical treatment. They could be questions about the types of treatment options available to you for the type of cancer you have or about the side effects or the necessity of the treatment.

Ask questions about all options and outcomes you have heard about. Ask questions about how to support your body during treatments being recommended. Go for a second opinion and even a third opinion, and ask the same questions. I discovered by going for a second opinion, that having surgery would have been ill-advised, since I had liver and lung metastases that needed more attention and removing the breast tumor would have not resulted in a cure. The first surgeon was insistent that I make an appointment immediately to have the mastectomy. I'm so grateful that I had the fortitude to refuse and to go for the second opinion.

Ask questions about pain management, especially non-pharmacological approaches to pain management. Ask questions to learn about how to support your arteries, veins, bones and nerves, and if they will be affected by chemo or radiation. Will treatment affect your brain and its function, and what should you be doing to support it during treatment? If the physician you are talking to cannot answer these questions, ask him or her who else you could consult to discuss your questions.

Focusing on enhancing your body's ability to heal itself while having medical treatment is one of the most important things to do. You owe it to yourself and your amazing body so it can return to its former self. You might think that having surgery, chemo and radiation are passive. They do not have to be. You were an active part of the decisions if you are reading this book before you committed to any treatment. If not, you have the ability to become active in the choices from now on. It is never too late to make a change to how you deal with your cancer treatment. I only read about the mind-body connection when I was almost finished with chemo and about to start radiation. I learned that I could use visualization to help the healing and used a visualization of a healing golden light entering my body during every radiation treatment. My skin held up remarkably well with no burning or cracking open, which was common at that time, according to the radiation therapist. I did the same when I started receiving very painful hormone blocking injections that felt like they were being delivered with a horse syringe. I visualized my immune cells getting a boost of power to help them block and prevent any cancer cell from feeding off any nutrient cancer cells would try to steal from my body. They were stealth ninjas catching cancer cells and cutting off their source of energy. The imagery I used dates me, but I'm sure that you can find imagery and visualizations that speak to your sense of purpose and amusement.

Wellness approaches

I asked you earlier what the equal and opposite reaction your body needs to embrace to beat cancer. We looked at what it is that you want and what treatment options are available to you. Now it is time to figure out how you get to wellness. There are some areas that we have not covered with regards to the regular behaviors that might have led to or supported the cancer. Let us look at those old habits. What do you put into your body that may not be good for you? Do you think there is a link with this habit and cancer? Are you willing to give the habit up? Are there exclusions you need to inititate?

You have to know what your heart is telling you and then decide what you are going to follow – your inner knowledge or your ego? In one of Dr. Siegel's books he tells a story of a 90-year-old who smoked a cigar a day, ate hamburgers regularly and drank whiskey. When asked how he had lived to such a good age and what he thought about his so-called bad habits, his reply was that he believed that if he absolutely loved everything he put into his body it would do him no harm. He had an unshakable belief in this. If you have a similarly strong belief, you don't have to change a thing. If your belief is even a little shaky, I question if continuing this habit is good for you.

What about hydration? Do you put enough water into your body every day? We are supposed to drink around 4 liters of water a day. Only pure water qualifies, not fizzy drinks, juices, coffee or other dehydrating drinks like alcohol; just water. I know that I was chronically dehydrated for many years. My reasoning was that I would eat rather than drink. When I learned that cancer prefers a dehydrated body and one that isn't well oxygenated, things started to change for me. Are you getting enough water and oxygen for your blood to do its job? Moving your body is a great way to increase your oxygen intake, and you have to develop the habit of drinking more water.

This might be a good place for you to look at your diet and the nutrients you receive to support your immune system. Eating is not just filling your belly, it is about nourishing your body and soul. Are you eating foods that are necessary for the needs of your body? Ask any immigrant what he or she misses most about being away from the place he or she calls home. It is most often food! Start a practice of loving the food that you eat, even if you have had to change things in your diet. This love affair we have for food can be used to nourish us back to health. What you put into your body and how it makes you feel is important in healing. Food is healing if you spend the time enjoying your meals. The medicinal benefits of diet can only be activated if seen as true nourishment and honored as such.

Jeanette Bronee', author of, *Eat to Feel Full,* had taught me that I was doing my body a huge disservice by eating while standing up over the kitchen counter. She pointed out that the most powerful message I was giving my body was that I didn't have time for it and that I wouldn't give feeding it the importance to sit down and be mindful with every bite. I think this is what the old man in Dr. Siegel's story was trying to say. Take your time to enjoy every moment of everything you consume and you will feel nourished beyond physical satisfaction. Eating mindfully empowers your body to savor food and to fortify itself using the nutrients. Food is a powerful tool against cancer. I am not a dietician, so that is probably all I can safely say about using diet as a weapon against cancer. There are many books written on the subject and there are superb coaches and nutritionists specializing in this field. Look for your food guide.

Adding a well thought out diet and supplements to protect you and to kill off cancer is an essential part of living life with cancer. The medical treatments are usually passive, but eating, drinking water and thinking are active fighting strategies. While you are getting rid of the cancer your diet is an active way for you to focus your energy towards denying cancer the space inside your body. Eat thoughtfully and mindfully with every bite and you will be "fighting cancer with your fork," as Kim Dalzell PhD says. Dr. Dalzell's book, *Challenge Cancer and Win,* has a chapter for each different type of cancer identifying the food that can help the body fight that specific cancer more effectively. I have to reiterate that I do not know what and if you will cure the cancer. The point of paying attention to your body is that your habits regarding your body must not continue to add doubt and fear to the equation. Take a conscientious and systematic approach to what you choose as support for your body and your body will become a force to stand up against cancer.

I have created a body worksheet you might find useful when thinking about all the aspects of your health and healing. You could use it for recording and tracking questions you want to ask healing professionals and to make commitments to hold yourself accountable for.

Body Worksheet

Challenge	Questions to ask	Commitment	Notes
e.g., Dehydration	Is it safe to drink lots of water during radiation?	Drink two more liters per day.	Doctor says it's safe to increase hydration - it protects kidneys.

Movement

I believe that getting out of bed and sitting in the chair when Eileen visited me was a symbolic act of my first movement after allowing myself to slip into despair the first time I had cancer. My inactivity one week after surgery was unlike me. More typical was my getting up to wash my hair three hours after surgery with a drain hanging from my armpit. During my hair washing, a visiting nun had come to see the new cancer patient (me) and couldn't hide her disapproval when she found that whom she had come to minister to was the woman bending over the hand basin,. She didn't stay after making it quite clear that I had wasted her time. That, and a couple of other experiences, formed the impressions of how a "good cancer patient" was meant to behave. It made me feel invalid and I resorted to hiding from the world until Eileen changed that expectation of myself. Since then, I have tried not to trap myself in an inactive state. Symbolically I see moving as equivalent to living. Later, when the second and third bouts of cancer happened, movement was a significant symbol of my taking the path towards healing.

By sharp contrast, the second time I was diagnosed, I had been working too hard for long hours and would flop down in front of the TV in the evenings after supper. After I was diagnosed with metastases in my liver and left lung, it was not easy to get up the energy to go outside and walk. I forced myself to because I believed that my life depended on it. All I could do the first time was to walk to the second driveway away from our house. While I walked, I created a mantra I stole from a song in an old musical, *South Pacific* , the chorus was - "I'm gonna wash that man right out of my hair" which I turned into "I'm gonna walk this cancer right out of my life."

It gave me a sense of purpose and determination, and eventually, when I was able to walk around the whole neighborhood, I did so with a huge grin on my face.

The third time I needed to get moving against cancer was when I was in the cardiology unit after cancer cells had been detected in the fluid around my heart and in my left lung. I was itching to go home but was told that I would have to stay until I got my blood pressure up and could tolerate my heart rate going up a certain amount without shortness of breath or chest pain. My silly daughters took this to heart and started walking me more and more briskly up and down the hospital hallway. I was wearing a heart monitor, which was hooked up to screens at the nurses' station, as well as ones above the doors of each patient room. I could see my heart rate and compare it with the other rates that showed up above and below mine. The girls used this as a cheerleading technique by commentating as though they were at a horse race. "Nearly beating number two, yes! Number one has beaten number two, now we see number one gaining on number five - the fastest in the race so far. Can number one catch up and win the race? YES!!" When I did, they let out an almighty cheer, because I had reached my target heart rate, was not only able to sustain that rate, but do so while laughing out loud with total joy for my accomplishment without triggering chest pain. The nurses who came out to see what the commotion was about were met with my daughters saying, "Oh, don't worry, she has cancer and we have been cheering her on." That got some shocked looks, but I had met the goal and was discharged later that day. Maybe it was because the doctors and nurses wanted to restore peace and quiet to their ward. You can tell that I am not an obedient patient.

My intention with writing this chapter was to give you some ideas to tackle the war in your head about your body and your possible disappointment in it. As I said earlier, you have done nothing wrong and neither has your body. The goal was to help you find things that you can believe in and nourish your body with. My daughter's showed me that there is strength in owning the cancer and how you manage it. I hope that you find the ability to do this too.

Now that you have ideas about what to seek when looking to support your body, we will tackle what to do about your spirit. Without your spirit you are nothing. Cancer may seem to break your spirit, but this is not a permanent state. You can find your spirit in the midst of the cancer turmoil. All you have to do is to consciously seek spirituality again.

SECTION 3

SPIRIT

Chapter 9

SPIRIT

———— ~ ————

In this chapter I will help you explore spirit and spirituality. For those of you who have strong faith already, you might not have as many struggles with this topic. Hopefully you will find some thoughts about how to make your daily practices a deeper experience with God and your soul in everything you do no matter what your faith background is.

Finding your soul and focusing on spirituality is the third key to fighting cancer. I'll show you ways that you can connect with your spirituality if you do not already have spiritual practices or if you have become disconnected with them. I have found from all my reading and learning about fighting cancer, success occurs when mind, body and spirit are included in the healing.

My impression of spirituality is less formal now, after many years of stumbling and stubbornness, so I will speak less of God and more about soul. I do believe that you have a spirit and that it is the essence of life. In order to live life fully, you cannot ignore this vital part of living. I have set out to give you some thoughts on how you can start spiritual practices that can reach that deep part of your being that yearns to be heard and nourished too. The obstacle to becoming more aware of your spirit or spirituality may be having cancer in the first place. The dull emptiness felt after being diagnosed blocks any endeavors at deep thought, let alone deep spiritual connection. With my first diagnosis I considered myself as being devout, and yet, I was totally unable to pray. Every time I tried to pray there was a void. I could not pray to a God I was angry with; my anger made me feel ashamed, so I avoided God. Anger, hurt and fear did not create a prayerful environment for me. All I could muster up was to pray for my children and those prayers were pretty feeble because I really didn't want God to see or hear me.

A place I found myself connecting with more than my corporal being was under a shady tree in my mother's garden. This pink pepper tree had a smell that reminded me of my childhood when I played under the big tree. Now it was an old, well-established tree with solid branches bigger than the bole of the tree I knew as a teenager. It was solid and sound. I leaned against the strong trunk, in the shade, surrounded by its smell and I wept. It was as though the tree understood and accepted me. It allowed me to pour all my thoughts, fears, desires and dreams into that space. While I was under the pepper tree, I didn't feel alone or abandoned. I felt supported and loved. You might think this is an odd way to start a chapter on spirituality, but this is where I was able to have a spiritual connection outside of myself again after my cancer diagnosis. It didn't have to be consciously with God. What I experienced that day was a connection with my soul deep inside me. Since then, trees have remained my strongest connection with God, the universe and my spirit.

I trust that you will find your connection because you know to seek it. Mine happened by accident.

Cancer can be a reminder that you have neglected your spirit. Contemporary lifestyles dictate a fast pace, short attention spans and little time to stop and be fully present in anything you do. You rush; spend little time doing anything that causes you to pause, so you neglect the most vital part of life - your soul. Even when you become aware of this, you carry on living your busy life, too busy to be grateful for what you have until it seems too late. Now you are diagnosed with cancer. That is when the guilt and self-deprecation starts: If only I had..... "Too late" can result in an enormous sense of despair. Your prayers at this time can feel desperate calls for help when you know that you have not been fully present for God or yourself so instead, as I did, you are shamed into retreat. Stop the rushing and not paying attention and start to place significance on spirituality and daily meditation time where nothing is done except trying to be.

What is this thing called the spirit or soul? This is not a religious question, just a philosophical one. When I was at medical school while training to become an occupational therapist, we had to do a full year of dissection on one cadaver for the entire year. The cadaver I shared with three other students was relatively young and in perfect physical condition. The cause of death was not revealed to us and we did not question it. What I did question was the difference between this perfect physical being lying inert on a dissection table and the live people moving around me. Why was he dead and why were they alive? What made that difference? There was no breath; there was no heartbeat, yet all the organs that could have been filled with air or should have been beating were intact and perfect. This is when I discovered the existence of something bigger than my comprehension, a mystery that led me to believe that the soul is a marvelously intriguing thing. It made me believe. Not to believe in a religion at that time, but in a way that stirred my own spirit to feel awe and humility in the face of this great secret of life. There was a spiritual difference between life and lifelessness. That was a deeply spiritual experience for me and I still think of that man with gratitude and reverence for what he revealed to me about life. It was my first real connection with God.

Vitality is a word that means life or relating to life. Vitality is described in the dictionary as the capacity for survival; the power to live. Our organs are called vital because they sustain life. When cancer interferes, I believe that you have to get to the core of your existence in order to live life fully again. That is a vital truth for me.

Finding your purpose

Man's universal search for meaning is the search for a greater sense of purpose in the world. People who belong to formal religions have a particular understanding of that purpose as understood and described by dogma. Spiritual practices are prescribed and taught and followers spend their lifetime perfecting their spiritual practices and rituals, all with the purpose of achieving their highest connection to God and to attain eternal life. Cancer offers an opportunity to deepen faith and spirituality.

I believe that everyone can attain spirituality and a deeper meaning to life, whether through religion or not. I also believe that it is important to seek purpose, especially because cancer forces questioning of the meaning of life. The diagnosis makes you face your mortality. Knowing your purpose is a way for you to navigate through the emotions and achieve a sense of peace again.

The purpose exercise I describe below is one that I do with all my leadership clients. I do this exercise with them because all exceptional leaders explain that having a clear purpose for what they do gives them the energy to face all the obstacles they know they will encounter in business. They also believe in having daily practices to strengthen their minds and spirit to give them the physical energy and fortitude they need to do their jobs well. Mind, body and spirit work together for health and vitality in business so why shouldn't it work when dealing with cancer? You might not be striving for world peace, but inner peace is just as important!

Finding your purpose exercise: Start with a blank piece of paper. Make a list of all your natural talents. These are things people identified in you from when you were growing up. What did they say about you regularly? Things that will remind you are things others said you were always doing or not doing, things they said you were good at and ways you interacted with people, objects and animals. For example, things people said about my father when he was growing up were that he was able to fix anything. He became an engineer and he was always inventing things to fix a problem. Add all the things you believe are your natural talents to this list.

Now make a list of the skills that you have gained through education, training or life.

Make a new list of all your values. Things that you value in life and things you won't live without. If you need help with this, go online and search the word "values." You will find a list of over a hundred. Choose the ones that are most meaningful to you. Look back at your lists and highlight the top two or three most important to you in each list.

Now complete this sentence: With these talents, skills and values (you can mention the top one or two of each), my purpose is to ____ (fill the blank) in the world. If the completed sentence excites you and makes you a little scared of its breadth, you probably have uncovered your real purpose. If the sentence diminishes your energy, you have not yet found the purpose that gives you meaning. Keep thinking about this and revisit this sentence often. Your purpose will reveal itself. It is your reason to live - your "why." Living your purpose every day with or without cancer is what gives meaning to life and connects you to the world with a deeper sense of belonging. People who have a formalized faith sometimes find this exercise easier. Spirituality gives a sense of faith in life and the worth of living. We have to know why life is worth living.

Spiritual practices

It is important to have spiritual practices that allow your mind to quieten and for you to listen to your hearts and souls. It helps to find ways to be and to live with purpose.

Spirituality is very personal, so do whatever you believe in. I experience my most spiritual moments when I am surrounded by nature. One of those experiences was when I visited the Redwood forests. The majesty of the ancient, enormous trees that dwarf humans moved me deeply. I was in awe as I stood in silence, admiring the greatness of the trees and the insignificance of my stature alongside them. I felt as though I was in a cathedral surrounded by light filtering through the branches. The sounds of the wind high up in the treetops, the sounds of the trees' slight movement were evidence of my witnessing living proof of endurance and fortitude beyond what I could imagine. Being there gave me strength and peace. Interestingly, most of the people I encountered in the forest seem to feel the same awe and chose to witness it in silence with me. The contrasts of the grandeur of the trees with the vulnerability of the delicate spider webs inside the folds of the bark reminded me of our coexistence in the world and moved me to a deep spiritual place. I used this experience as a visualization when I needed a place of healing years later.

Another spiritual experience I often draw on is from a photograph taken in a nature reserve in Brazil. At the base of the stem of a huge tree was a fragile mushroom with a stem as thin as a thread and a top part of the mushroom much bigger than the stem should be able to support. The impossibility of the biomechanics of this mushroom's existence and ability to remain upright fascinated me. It drew me in and I stared at the photograph for ages. It moved my soul. The impossible is possible when we believe. If we pay attention in nature, we see evidence of impossibility becoming possible over and over. This is where I find my most spiritual moments.

Music can have that effect on you as well. It can help you feel connected to something beyond what you are experiencing in any one moment and elevate your mood. It has the ability to move you emotionally and spiritually. The first time I heard Pachelbel's *Canon in D*, I had that experience. Smetana's *Moldau* still transports me to a vivid scene of a brook in a forest, no matter where I find myself. Find music that does that for you and add it to your visualization.

Musicians and composers are aware of the powerful spirituality of a chord, a flat or sharp, the sound of the double bass or cello, oboe or flute, and the full volume of a pipe organ. Baroque music has been found to elicit healing responses in the brain. Operas sung in foreign languages continue to mesmerize and move people emotionally across the world. Music touches our souls in marvelously healing ways. Seek what moves your soul. Your body will feel the benefits.

Deep spiritual experiences help put life back into perspective. It gives you peace of mind and a sense that you belong and are an important part of the world. Sometimes feeling insignificant and humble can make you feel grateful for where you are and what you're experiencing - even when the experience is cancer. Cancer can be a great teacher of life, even when you don't want to admit it.

Sometimes it is impossible to connect with your soul or to feel spiritual. It is important to find a way to shift into a spiritual place regularly when living with cancer. It is an essential coping mechanism and a vital healing practice. How to do so at will is something that you can learn to do. Even deeply religious people will tell you that they are not always able to achieve a deep spiritual experience every time that they pray. It takes practice. But, as the old Irish man said to the priest who asked him what he did in church every day, "Sometimes I sits and prays and sometime I just sits." Sometimes you can shift gears into spirituality; sometimes not. Sometimes just sitting is enough; embrace that as a spiritual state of being.

Having daily practices are helpful. Buddhist priests take years to be able to reach a deep state of meditation at will. Contemplative prayer takes practice. In church they do not teach contemplative prayer, they teach active asking prayers. Ask for forgiveness, ask for help, ask for a cure. Spiritual prayer is silently sitting in the presence of God in a meditative state, focusing on nothing more than your breath. Buddhists teach focus on the breath in and breath out as the core of practicing meditation. Teachers of Christian contemplative prayer also use breathing with a mantra involving Jesus to teach deep prayer. A technique I was taught by a nun years ago was to breathe Jesus in and to breathe the stress or fear out. When I was fighting cancer, I turned the mantra into breathing in healing and breathing out the cancer.

I recently came across the "release" meditation, taught by Brendon Burchard, where you repeat the word "release" with each breath; this could be apt when dealing with cancer. Dr. Dispenza teaches a meditation called *Changing Two Beliefs and Perceptions.* There are many YouTube videos to learn from. Searching for the release meditation is something you can start doing right now.

Here is a relaxation practice that I have taught many people to use in order to quieten their minds and to learn to be still.

Sit or lie quietly and focus on your breathing. When your mind fills with a thought, acknowledge the thought and let it go; it will come back if it is important, so let it go. Go back to the breath. There are no demands other than to breathe. There are no prescriptions to say you should do this for one minute or 30 minutes. Just sit and breathe to practice. Put the book aside right now, take in a deep breath and allow your eyes to close as you breathe out. Now just sit there and feel the breath go in and come out. It isn't important if you focus on the feeling of the breath around your nose or if you feel it raise and lower your chest or abdomen. Link your mind to the breath any way that you can and fix your consciousness on your breath.

Sit like that for as long as you can. If you get an itch, let it go and go back to the breath. Don't get annoyed or impatient with yourself. Everyone struggles with major thought interruptions, body sensations, itches, aches and pains at first. Just allow yourself to bring your focus back to the breath. It really doesn't matter if you manage to sit there having focused on five breaths or for five minutes. The fact that you were willing to start practicing is what is a gift to yourself; an investment into your spirit so you can be more effective reducing the power that cancer has over you. Be patient with yourself, but start. It isn't about perfection; it is about making a start.

Once you have made a start you might identify things that you need to help you limit distractions while meditating. These could be sounds, smells or practices. Try several out and see what helps you the most.

When I started trying to meditate, a friend of mine sent me some nature recordings that I found very helpful. One in particular was called the dawn chorus. It was a recording of birds awakening in the very early morning, starting with small chirps and calls, replies to the calls and eventually the very vibrant sounds of the morning when out in the bush in South Africa. This recording was one that worked for me in the background when I was trying to get into a meditative state. Another recording among the ones my friend sent me was the sound of the ocean. She found that one particularly soothing; I did not. It disrupted my sense of calm every time I heard a wave crashing on rocks and it made me feel more anxious. I loved being at the beach and was always very energetic and active either body surfing or exploring the rock pools. When a wave came you had to be ready to react! Sounds of the ocean waves are too busy for a meditation for me.

Buddhists sometimes tap a small, melodious bell to help them reach their deeper state of meditation. Lighting a delicately fragrant candle or incense stick helps people as well. Again, these were too distracting for me; my mind would conjure up dreams and memories attached to the smells that would divert my attention. Try it out for yourself with your favorite candle. If you have a connection with an aroma that relaxes you, it will be an effective way to set the tone for your meditative state.

Many authors and teachers use guided imagery to help people to get into a deep meditative state. Dr. Siegel uses the "special place" visualization. Once you are able to get to your special place with a clear picture of what it looks, smells, feels and sounds like, you are invited to remain there in silence. You can add the words, "This is a place where my body is efficient and effective in restoring itself; this is a place where my mind and soul are at peace. This is a place where I can be whole." Then just be there with your breath. The visualization helps to get you into a calmer, more silent mind space before you enter into meditation.

Here is another way to still the busy mind. It is progressive relaxation technique and goes like this: Start off sitting or lying in a comfortable upright or stretched out posture. Take a few deep breaths and close your eyes. Now start saying a short word like "peace." When I do this with clients I use a neutral word like "one." Repeat the word at whatever pace initially comes to you - one, one, one. Now consciously slow the pace of your word - one....one....one. Continue to repeat the word a few more times - one......one......one......one.

Take your mind outside the room you are in and search for a sound outside. If the sound moves away, find a new sound. Return to your word - one........one.........one. Now search for a sound inside the room you are in. Attach your mind to that sound for a while. Return to your word -

one........one.........one.......one. Continue to repeat the word at this pace while you do a slow scan of your body like this: Feel the muscles of your face and head, consciously relax the muscles of your lips, cheeks and jaw. One.....one.....one.

Become aware of your neck, relax your neck and let the tension go from your neck, allowing it to comfortably settle into a good posture. One......one.........one. Move your attention to your shoulders. Allow them to drop away from your head. Feel your shoulder blades relax back and you're still saying your word. One........one......one. Let your arms become heavy and relaxed from your shoulders, through your elbows, wrists and fingers. Allow your fingers to fall open gently. One.......one.......one. Become aware of your back and allow it to relax from between your shoulders, mid back and low back. Feel the support your back is receiving from the chair or bed. Go back to your word - one......one........one.

Become aware of your chest as it rises and falls with your breath. Relax the muscles of your chest and you're still saying your word. One....one.....one. Now focus on your stomach. Allow all the tension to flow out of the muscles as you feel your stomach relax. Back to your word - one.....one...one.

Move your attention to your hips. Let your pelvis, your muscles around your hipbones, the muscles of your buttocks relax; allow your legs to roll outwards comfortably. One....one...one. Pay attention to your thighs front and back and allow your muscles to relax all the way down to your knees. One...one....one. Become aware of the muscles below your knees, down to your ankles. Relax your knees and ankles and feel the support your feet are given by the floor or feel the sides of your ankles supported by the bed. Let all the tension go. One...one....one.

Your whole body is relaxed and supported, your mind is quietly repeating your word, your breathing is slow and steady. This is a safe place where your body is ready to heal itself. Your immune system is perfect and doing its job effortlessly. Stay there and focus only on your breath for a while. When you are ready, start becoming aware of your word again - one, one, one.

Now search for a sound outside your room. Bring your attention back to this room and search for a sound, gently opening your eyes and becoming aware of the light and shapes in this room. You have brought your peacefulness and healing back into this room with you. Take a deep breath in and out, stretch your whole body and you are ready to face the rest of the day and the world fully present and connected.

Flag these pages and use these practices to help you start your meditative explorations. You can introduce God into the meditative part with you being present in His golden, healing light.

You might want to make a recording of the relaxation described above. If you record it on your phone you can listen to it with your own voice at any time. I have used the word visualization to describe this exercise and it can also be referred to as guided imagery. There is a slight difference between guided imagery and visualization. Technically, visualization is creating pictures through words or by thinking about a specific place visually. Some people struggle with being able to see pictures, so a guided imagery might work better. A guided imagery can be a conversation rather than a picture that you create in your imagination. Either way, they elicit real physiological responses that promote healing.

Living with purpose helps you identify the contribution you want to make in the world and it helps you to see how you can accomplish that. Making a contribution means giving. When you have cancer, you suddenly become the recipients of pity, sympathy, attention and even charity. It stings. You can change that by starting to look outwards. Who can you give to? Who needs you in the world and what does the world need from you? Altruism has been shown by brain scientists to immediately create connections between people. Showing empathy, even just feeling empathy for another individual creates a cellular connection outside of your brain with another human being's brain through your mirror neurons. These are real cells that can be seen firing up on functional MRIs (fMRI). Adding generosity and benevolence to a thought about an individual could change the life of someone you encounter without using words.

A familiar line in the Ella Wheeler Wilcox *Solitude poem* is:

Laugh, and the world laughs with you;
Weep, and you weep alone.
In another verse she says:
Succeed and give, and it helps you live.

Yesterday my youngest daughter, Sarah-Jane and I had an encounter with two homeless men that made me reflect on our overall disconnection with others as social beings. Sarah-Jane smiled at the man as he asked for some change. I made eye contact with the other man. We had no change to offer, but they remarked how much they appreciated us acknowledging them and their existence. They showed genuine happiness for our acknowledgement alone. In that moment we had made their lives better, even though we had no money. We had made a connection.

This is so true when dealing with the cancer diagnosis. We are alone in our thoughts, fears and suffering, but when we share a moment of joy with another human being, we connect to the world and its heartbeat. We need people and we need a spiritual connection to them.

Daniel Goleman, famous for his multiple books on emotional intelligence, relates an experiment done on a busy subway station platform. The time was peak commuter travel time. A man wailed and shred his clothing, showing extreme distress, begging for attention, but the busy commuters rushed by without stopping or paying attention. This happened over and over as trains arrived and left. No one reached out to the man. Did no one have compassion? Goleman found that as long as people remain preoccupied with their activities and needs, rushing along, oblivious of others, behavior remains devoid of empathy and we cannot influence the world around us for good.

After several trials of the experiment, one person made eye contact with the distressed, wailing man and consciously felt compassion towards him. Immediately the crowd of commuters appeared to become aware of the man and surrounded him, trying to understand his language and find out what caused his distress. No words were initially spoken, just a conscious connection and empathy. This empathy from one individual was enough to trigger the mirror neurons in the brains of many people around the man and immediately changed their behavior towards him.

I think this is a powerful example of how our thoughts can be our connection with others—our spirit connecting outside of ourselves for the good of mankind.

A thought of kindness from you towards another person while waiting for your treatment or test in the same room could make a big difference to his/her level of hope. I try to keep this in mind when I see people in the infusion room at my oncologist's office. The people around me do not have to know that I am feeling for them. I try to do this by thinking encouraging thoughts like, "Look at what a strong and dignified person you are while having your treatment, which I know isn't easy."

Goleman says that if you acknowledge another person's strength, identify with him or her for his or her ultimate success and send him or her your love, his or her spindle cells will receive your message, light up in the brain, as seen on a fMRI, and give the person a sense of wellbeing. Remember that the mind can trigger the release of endorphins and encephalin, which trigger relaxation and stimulate your immune system into efficiency. On top of that, you are lifting the spirits of the person you share your intentions with and your own soul sings.

Did you know that you can pass the gift of healing on with your thoughts? You do now and it is a powerful gift. Share it generously. It will help you fight cancer in the world around you. You will start your own healing movement!

Prayer and a shared purpose is a powerful way to share spirituality in a group or community. I recently interviewed the son of a woman who was diagnosed with a brain tumor. He was doing mission work thousands of miles away when he heard the news. All he was able to do for his mother was to pray. It helped him and it gave him peace of mind that he was able to do something meaningful from so far away. When he got home, their community gathered to pray as well, and they all believe that his mother's surgery was successful and that she started to improve as a result.

This chapter was a tricky one to write, but one that showed you that you can find ways to deepen your existing faith and relationship with God or start conscious daily practices to connect with your spirit in a new way with deeper meaning. My beliefs are my personal understanding of spirituality. You will have your own understanding about the topic. The bottom line is that you need to learn to fortify your mind and that leads directly to deepening your spirituality, in my opinion. My experience is that you cannot overcome cancer in a void. You are mind, body and spiritual being, so you have to learn how to reconnect with your spirit and with others in very deep and meaningful ways in order to feel that your life is fulfilled. The practices shared are my favorite ones. I'm sure, as you explore this aspect of your healing, you will come across ones that are most meaningful to you. You have a good starting point now. Grow and develop your spirituality consciously.

I have said throughout the book that you need partners in this quest to heal from cancer. The next chapter will look at ways to select the right support and to teach your significant cancer warriors or important allies what meaningful things they can do to support you in living your life. Skattie once said that it is our families and closest friends who are the real heroes in cancer. I know that she is right, so believe that you need to support them in supporting you with clear direction.

SECTION 4

SUPPORT

Chapter 10

YOUR SUPPORT SYSTEM

The trouble when you have been diagnosed with cancer is that everyone wants to help somehow, but they do not know how. They are as lost as you are and often afraid to admit it. In this chapter I'll explore the value of having people there to support you, to do specific tasks, to listen and sometimes just to be with you. I do not know that you consciously define roles and responsibilities to your friends and family in general, however having cancer changes that. I think that a conscious plan with and for your family and friends gives them a way to process what is happening in your lives with cancer and to contribute to your wellness journey.

How to deal with this is for you to explain what you need from people around you. Everyone in your support team will be different; you cannot expect the same from everyone, so it takes some work to figure out what each person is good at and how that can help you in your success journey. It may take a little time to figure out how each person can help, but once you know what you want from each person, you need to educate him or her so that each one can be the best support person for the thing that he or she is good at.

I have a friend, Marsha, who did so much for me when I had few local friends and I felt that I didn't want to burden my daughters with the daily fears and anxieties, thoughts and feelings. Marsha read me like a book and I think she intuitively really knew what I needed when I didn't. Yet she was the one to ask me how she could best support me. She wasn't afraid to admit that she didn't know what I might need and was also willing to ask. I didn't really know what I wanted but Marsha came along for the ride anyway. She didn't get frustrated or impatient with me, she was like a rock; steadfast and silent but she didn't allow me to wallow or take myself too seriously either. She would nudge me along with her humor and knew what buttons to push to get me out of inactivity or from slipping out of good habits. One of the things I loved about her was that she would remind me of the bag of healthy "sticks and twigs" I carried around with me when she saw that I was being tempted to eat sugar or unhealthy food. This meant so much to me, and as I write this, I realize that I have not thanked her properly for the wonderful friend she has been. People who really love us have endless generosity and are vital in our recovery.

CHOOSE

~

You have to be discerning about who you surround yourself with. I told you the story about PD. On the surface she appeared to everyone to care so much, but her behavior created a caustic environment for Liz and myself. We had to make a conscious effort to avoid PD. I think it would have been easier to say something. At the time, I wasn't as discerning as I became later.

Sometimes your most significant relationships could be the most toxic. When I was halfway through the radiation, having completed chemo, my husband found me crying on our balcony. I was afraid and sad, struggling to see a good outcome for the treatment and an end to cancer. All I wanted was for him to hold me close and to tell me that things would be OK again. He couldn't. He was dealing with his own fear of losing me, held me at arm's length and told me that he had to start distancing himself from me because of that. That moment stayed with me for a very long time. It did help me recognize that I had to find the strength to survive on my own. Skattie entered my life at the right time to help me find the strength and to give me the support that I needed to survive. Without her, I do not think I could have made it through the first fight with cancer.

By the time of the second diagnosis, my marriage had become empty. In spite of having endured immigration together, the relationship had not improved. Skattie had passed away many thousand miles away. I was aware that new fear, loneliness and resentment were eating me up inside, creating a fertile internal field for cancer. I knew that I had to move out of the marriage if I wanted to survive but the thought terrified me. Living with a combination of fear and resentment became an even bigger burden. My wholeness coach, Jeanette, helped me look at all aspects of toxins and nourishment in my life. She questioned where I saw myself succeeding and where in my life there were obstacles. Gently, she helped me face the reality of my resentment and how it would not let me move forward towards a cure. I knew deep inside me that I had to make a very bold move and leave my marriage, even though I cowered at the thought.

It took the support of all my daughters and my dear friend, Marsha, to find the courage to leave. Separating from my marriage was hard but it gave me the freedom to start rebuilding the trust I had lost in myself. It gave me the ability to focus on fighting cancer head-on with a less conflicted emotional environment. I started focusing on restoring my faith in myself and began the true healing that I needed.

You need people around you who make you feel safe, who you have the utmost trust in and who you are certain accept you as you are. Not because you satisfy their need to be a caregiver, but because they genuinely care about you.

Think about the types of support that you need and want. Make a list. If I were to write the list now, mine would include:

- Someone who would be able to give me emotional support for the dark, as well as the good days
- Someone who was rational and efficient to do research about treatment, diet, supplements and useful tips
- Someone to laugh with and be totally relaxed with and who would lift my spirits
- Someone to push me and keep me on track

You might find all these characteristics in one person or in several people. I would identify characteristics in my family members that could meet my needs and ask them to be that support for me. I did a little of this with two of my daughters who were living with me when I became ill the third time. They became my researchers, shoppers, cooks and companions to medical appointments. When it became too much with the endless appointments, they delegated this to another daughter. It helps to spread the duties so that the people who support you with more regular, daily activities do not become fatigued or burnt out.

Outside support can be very helpful for the everyday tasks that are less intimately linked to your emotions and healing. You could have one of your trusted supporters vet the caregivers for you.

Having a close friend and support is a godsend. In the absence of that intimate support, your journal can fill that void for you.

WHAT TO LOOK FOR

The chief characteristic of the people on your support team who you want close to you is that they accept you inside and out. They know you and have loved you for who you are and will be there to reflect your best self as you go through this experience, no matter what. People who are steadfast and reliable with their mood and acceptance of you are people who you want in the intimate core of your support. The things about their personality and behavior that you know doesn't change, is what makes them trusted. When you do turn to them for advice or to run ideas by them, you know that you can rely on honesty about what they think; always with your best interests in mind. Surround yourself with people like this and with people who are consistently like this. They are always the same, so you can trust their moods and behavior to be what they have always been when you are with them. Erratic people are not a good choice for now. You need stability now, since there is enough turmoil for you to deal with. People who are generally calm are good additions to the group of supporters. Sometimes we need cheerleaders who are loud and will jostle us along; sometimes we need people who have a calming effect on us. These are people who can be helpful when you are trying to practice your visualizations and relaxation techniques.

People who love you, warts and all, are the best. These are friends who have experienced life with you or those you know you want to experience life with. They are patient, strong, trustworthy with your emotions and don't fall for your brand of BS. They will call you out when you are slacking off and making excuses. They will hug you and hold you and have a good cry with you when life dishes up the hard stuff. Some know intuitively what it is that you need, but they will still want your guidance to reassure them that what they can and do give is enough and on point.

People to avoid are people who are self-focused. They show up more bereft than you about the cancer. Your parents will be truly distressed but that is not what I'm talking about. These self-focused people surprise you and others with how your cancer affects them. If they are unable to put their feelings aside and be there for you, they will drain your energy and that of your real supporters.

Beware also of the person who is very opinionated about latest trends, news articles they have read and their experiences with other people's cancer. Their constant advice for what you should or shouldn't be doing, eating or taking, which doctor you should be seeing instead of your own, which treatment center you should be going to is exhausting. They do not honor your decisions and will have an endless stream of solutions you should pay attention to.. Avoid people who "should" on you. Period. You have to set boundaries and be firm about your solid faith in the choices that you have made and politely request that they do not offer you advice that makes you doubt what you are doing.

Chatty people can also be exhausting. They fill every silence, have to tell you everything about most things you do not find as fascinating as they think you should and can literally wear you down. Fighting cancer is hard work physically and mentally. You do not have the bandwidth to deal with so much information, especially when it is not relevant or pertinent. Politely listening is an encouragement for more input from this type of person. Here again, boundaries can be helpful. You might have a trusted supporter help you do this for you. You cannot have your energy drained by the exuberance the other person has for topics they find sensational and newsworthy. Here is an example of what I am referring to.

I was sitting in the chemo infusion room at my oncologist's office a while ago and "Chatty Cathy" sat opposite me, bending the ear of her friend who was having chemo. The chairs were close to each other, so the woman having chemo in the next chair who had been trying to work on her computer was regaled with the same stories. I was only there for about 15 minutes but in that time I had heard three stories of people Chatty Cathy knew of who had been diagnosed with cancer. One was a real trooper but she wasn't doing so well because she had a rare incurable type of cancer for which chemo wasn't working. The next person she spoke about was a man who worked with another friend. He was so ill with chemo they had to stop his treatment to have blood transfusions and even with the transfusions he is anemic, so they might not carry on with the chemo. Poor man, who knows what will happen to him. And then there was her neighbor a few streets over whose mother is dying of cancer; so sad. How I didn't scream out loud I do not know. The woman on the left kept sighing loudly and stared at her computer, visibly uncomfortable with these stories. Cathy's friend just nodded and said things like "Oh" and "That's sad." This was all taken as encouragement for Cathy to dredge up another story of the suffering that cancer causes and the entertainment it obviously provided her. Boundaries!

This might be a good place to write in your journal about the boundaries you want to set around your space, your silence and your expectations for support during important times.

BE EXPLICIT ABOUT HOW
TO SUPPORT YOU

———— ～ ————

What was the purpose that you established for yourself in life? How will you accomplish that every day by living your life with the support from the people who you care about and those who care about you? Make a list of things that will make this journey succeed. To know what success looks like you have to be clear about what the outcome of this experience will be first.

Complete these sentences:

I will feel that I have succeeded to beat this cancer when ....

I need support to accomplish this by having someone to ....

You can repeat either of these sentences for every aspect of your life, for example, to:

- Do research into things to help your body, mind, spirit
- Attend my appointments with me
- Shop for healthy food options
- To help me visualize

And so on.

My healing team will help support me in finding a cure that works for me by ....

Once you have written down everything that comes to mind about what you need from your teams, you have to make a commitment to yourself about how you will use and be part of this healing. Write it down. For example:

My own commitment is to practice ....be diligent with.......... to seek support and help when I need it and guide my supporters so we all succeed.

The last thing to do here is to get each person on your team to accept the role you have given him or her and to ask for a commitment to be there for you in that role.

I just helped you explore how to bring meaning to the contributions your support team can make to help you through cancer. I also discussed how you can request things you need from them without feeling like they should already know or that they would figure it out. By the time you have reached this part of the book you will have created some ideas about what it means to you to have to live through cancer and beyond. You will hopefully have found comfort in finding out that you are not alone in your emotions, feelings or lack thereof. You have joined a special class of people, albeit unwillingly, but special we are. There is something precious about the wisdom and revelations about ourselves that we uncover through having been diagnosed with cancer.

None of us chose this; however, now that you are here and are surviving every day, you can look at this experience with completely new perspectives. I hope that I have helped the development of your perspectives about life and its importance to you. It is my hope that reading this book has helped you achieve some peace around cancer and that you have established your life's purpose and drive to live life fully.

CONCLUSION

I set out to write a book about healing and hope for people who have received a diagnosis of cancer. The fears and threats that live in your head and your heart forever now could make you not want to carry on. The realities of the cancer can make it hard to see any healing for you. Don't let that limit your beliefs in your ability to live a wonderful life of giving and loving for as long as you are able. I have said this already: Life is terminal; you know that you were born and that you will die. Like the cliché of the inscription on the headstone on a grave - it is the dash between the birthdate and death date that matters. What will you "dash" be like?

I believe that as long as you give to others and share your love whenever you can, life will be rich. I also believe that living intentionally with purpose and faith in the healing power of your mind, body and spirit you can overcome cancer. I believe that if you let people in and help them contribute to the richness of your journey, you will have the resources to give to others and to add richness to other lives you may not have encountered if it had not been for cancer.

I do not proclaim a prescription for a cure, but I do believe in healing. Healing can be arriving at a peaceful acceptance of what life has for you and it can be an avid fight to make your life better and to kick cancer out of your cells. It is an unwelcome guest, so I cannot tolerate it being there.

Cancer has taught me that I do not give up easily. I can see my future clearly ahead of me as a result of not having a future I could take for granted. I have a goal to receive my doctorate at the age of 80. That means that I have a lot more living to do, so cancer, move over and don't try to stop me!

I have read books about the brain and the mind, and the powerful tool it is in changing your internal environment. This insight has helped me believe that it is possible to cure cancer. It all starts with a decision about what you really want and what you are prepared to invest physically, mentally and spiritually in that decision. It will take effort and energy and it will be a full time endeavor. So is life.

A life lived alone is an unfulfilled life. Cancer is easier to beat with a strong support team. Keep looking around for the right people to be on your team. Start to live, love and don't forget to laugh. As you assemble your support, journal what and who you are looking for, what you want from them and what you will contribute to the world around you. Filling the pages of your journal is enriching and can fulfill a spiritual need as well.

I have shared what I know; now it is up to you. Go and live life loudly, mind, body, spirit and fully supported.

I raise my glass to you in celebration and encouragement.

L'Chaim! To Life!

ABOUT THE AUTHOR

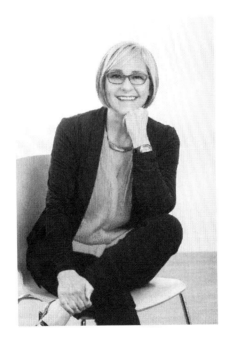

Lyn Cikara is a three-time metastatic breast cancer survivor, mother of five daughters, occupational therapist, leadership consultant, and South African American. She is passionate about empowering people to be their best, live life well and to see a future of hope beyond cancer.

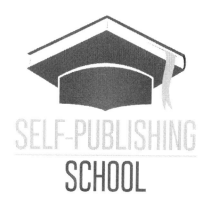

SCHOOL

NOW IT'S YOUR TURN

Discover the EXACT 3-step blueprint you need to become a bestselling author in 3 months.

Self-Publishing School helped me, and now I want them to help you with this FREE VIDEO SERIES!

Even if you're busy, bad at writing, or don't know where to start, you CAN write a bestseller and build your best life.

With tools and experience across a variety niches and professions, Self-Publishing School is the only resource you need to take your book to the finish line!

DON'T WAIT

Watch this FREE VIDEO SERIES now, and
Say "YES" to becoming a bestseller:

https://xe172.isrefer.com/go/sps4fta-vts/bookbrosinc2563

Made in the USA
San Bernardino, CA
28 April 2018